# ALTITUDE ILLNESS
## PREVENTION & TREATMENT

How to Stay Healthy At Altitude:
From Resort Skiing to Himalayan Climbing

**STEPHEN BEZRUCHKA M.D., M.P.H.**

THE
MOUNTAINEERS

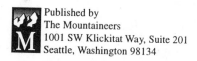 Published by
The Mountaineers
1001 SW Klickitat Way, Suite 201
Seattle, Washington 98134

First printing 1994, second printing 1996, revised 1998

Published simultaneously in Great Britain by Cordee, 3a DeMontfort Street,
Leicester, England, LE1 7HD

Manufactured in the United States of America

Edited by Maureen O'Neill
Design and typesetting by The Mountaineers Books

Library of Congress Cataloging-in-Publication Data
Bezruchka, Stephen.
      Altitude illness: prevention and treatment / Stephen Bezruchka.
                    p.      cm.
      Includes bibliographical references and index.
      ISBN 0-89886-402-X
  1. Mountain sickness. 2. Altitude, Influence of. I. Title.
RC103.A4B49  1994
606.9'893—dc20
                                              94-23111
                                              CIP

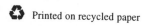 Printed on recycled paper

*To those who died of altitude illness*

# Contents

# Preface

"I get high with a little help from my friends," sang the Beatles, in the spirit of the sixties. Today more and more people want to get high, and they usually do it with friends, but they do it by ascending the world's highest peaks. The euphoria that comes with gaining altitude has been known to the Europeans for centuries. Upon attaining a summit, several of my German friends would say "und now we enjoy the high altitude." The heights are to be savored, but it is easy to get sick there too.

This portable book is designed to travel to altitude with you. Use it to:
• prepare for going to altitude.
• recognize the symptoms of acute mountain sickness.
• assess altitude-related problems accurately.
• decide on treatment methods.
• prevent serious consequences.

The information presented here is suitable for skiers, climbers, hikers, and trekkers heading to international destinations such as Quito, Ecuador; Lhasa, Tibet; Everest Base Camp; or high altitude sites in the U.S., such as Mount McKinley or Mammoth Mountain, California. Both the novice going to altitude for the first time and the seasoned hiker or climber will find this book an essential piece of gear.

Most treatments and medical advice suggested in this book are not FDA approved. Altitude illness is a nascent area of study that does not allow large controlled clinical trials for a number of reasons. One of the main obstacles lies in the fact that the illness affects relatively small numbers of people idiosyncratically. Secondly, high-altitude terrain makes research difficult. When far from expert help and facilities, use the information presented here to make the best of a difficult situation. Don't consider any drug treatments for altitude illness without first discussing them with a knowledgeable doctor and verifying drug dosages and indications.

# Acknowledgments

Many people helped me to craft the presentation of this material, provided new insights, and laboriously edited the drafts. Years ago Dr. Elaine Jong asked me to talk to her travel medicine audience on altitude illness. Then she and Dr. Marty Wolfe encouraged me to write on this topic. I appreciate the assistance of Dr. Herb Hultgren, one of the pioneers in the study of altitude illness. Dr. David Shlim contributed valuable ideas gleaned from his years of experience in Nepal. Drs. Buddha Basnyat, Penny Dawson, Tom Dietz, Jim Duff, Jim Litch, Mark Rabold, Brownie Schoene, and Yvonne Vaucher contributed their insight. Frances Klatzel, Bill Liske, and the staff at REI Adventure Travel, including Frith Maier and Rusty Brennan, helped me understand the guide's perspective and kept my language farther away from medispeak. Maureen O'Neill reminded me that clear, concise English is as important as the accuracy of the material presented. Thank you all.

The book has been updated in 1998, and includes useful sources of information on the Internet.

# How to Use This Book

Before a trip, read the whole book, and decide which drugs mentioned here you need to carry. During a trip, if you suspect you or your companion have altitude illness and need to assess the situation, turn to Chapter 4 and follow the steps to diagnose a specific disorder. A new term is italicized the first time it is used, and it is listed in the glossary.

# Chapter 1. Adapting to High Altitude

As you gain altitude, the air gets thinner, the pressure is lower, and less oxygen is available in the atmosphere. Imagine traveling in a modern pressurized airplane at 29,000 feet (8,800 m). If the cabin were to suddenly lose pressure, so that the air inside was at the same pressure as the air outside, you would lose consciousness and die in about four minutes unless you were breathing supplemental oxygen. However, Everest, at the same altitude, has been climbed many times without supplemental oxygen. What's the difference between the two scenarios? A gradual process called *acclimatization,* during which the body slowly gets used to lower levels of oxygen in the air. Individuals who have acclimatized properly are able to climb unassisted to extremely high altitudes and survive for short periods of time.

What happens as your body gets used to less oxygen? The end result of acclimatization, which occurs over a period of days to weeks, is that the body adapts to the increasingly rarefied air and delivers the necessary amounts of oxygen to the cells. The examples in this book describe the changes occurring in a person who is born and raised near sea level and who occasionally goes to altitude. Those who are born and raised at high altitudes, such as in the Himalaya or the Andes, may not experience these specific changes. If you live at moderate altitudes, such as at 5,000 feet (1,500 m) or more, you will find it easier to tolerate higher altitudes because you have already acclimatized, to some extent.

The following analogy is helpful in understanding the process of acclimatization. Imagine a freight train delivery system. Your blood vessels are the tracks. The train (your blood) is propelled by a locomotive (the heart) and has boxcars (your red blood cells) carrying a cargo (oxygen). The train's cargo is filled by a loader (your lungs) and empties its load at the factory (muscles, heart, brain, and other tissues) where the cargo is needed. Not all the cargo arriving at the loader at any one time is loaded. Much is sent back out, only to arrive again.

As an individual gains altitude, less and less cargo arrives at the loader each minute, but the demand at the factory remains constant. What does your body do? It responds by increasing the speed of the loader (makes the lungs breathe faster), increasing the speed of the train (makes the heart beat faster), and increasing the number of boxcars (makes more red blood cells). In this chapter, we will look at this process in detail.

In this book, *low altitude* is defined as 7,000 feet (2,100 m) or lower; *intermediate altitude* extends to 12,000 feet (3,660 m); *extreme altitude* is above 18,000 feet (5,500 m). The term *high altitude* encompasses the ranges of intermediate and extreme altitude.

## Breathing Adaptation

The most important adaptation you'll notice is the need to breathe more often. For example, when you drink from a water bottle you may need to stop in the middle to take a breath. Or you may need to stop talking to breathe. In general you'll breathe more both when active and when resting.

Each individual responds to the lowered oxygen at altitude differently. Some people breathe more often than others. Using the train analogy, if there is less oxygen in each loader (your lungs), then you will make the loader work faster in order to get the oxygen you need. Your capacity to do this can be decreased by taking sleeping pills, or increased by drugs, such as acetazolamide, which signal the loader to work faster. While some people advise using different techniques to increase your rate of breathing, simply breathing more, consciously or not, is the most important factor. Generally speaking, most world-class altitude climbers increase their breathing at altitude more than superb marathon runners do, likely due to different genetic makeup. However, psychological drive can make up for differences in the capacity to breath at altitude. An excellent example is provided by Peter Habeler and Reinhold Messner, the first two people to climb Everest without oxygen. One has a brisk rapid breathing response to altitude, while the other doesn't.

## Pulse Increase

Just as your respiration rate increases as you climb higher, your resting pulse increases during the first few days at altitude. If there is less oxygen in each boxcar (red blood cell), then the train's locomotive (your heart) will have to go faster to unload the same amount of oxygen at the factory as before.

It's a good idea to measure your pulse rate each day when you are resting and relaxed at an altitude destination. You can take your pulse in bed, before you go to sleep, but taking it immediately after awakening in the morning is probably better.

As you become more acclimatized, you will notice that your pulse drops, and there is less pounding in your chest. This can be a sign that your body is responding well to altitude. Drugs for angina or for high blood pressure may limit this response, in which case taking your pulse won't be a useful way to judge what is happening. Such drugs include beta blockers (atenolol, metoprolol, propranolol, timolol), calcium channel blockers (verapamil, diltiazem, nifedipine), and digoxin.

## Urinary Response

The body performs a diuresis at altitude; that is, you urinate more and get rid of fluids. If the freight train represents your blood, then diuresis means getting rid of non-cargo carrying cars, such as empty flat beds. Diuresis occurs when you sleep at 10,000 feet (3,050 m) or higher, and is thought to occur through stretch receptors in the heart. When diuresis takes place, you will notice having to get up at night to urinate one or two times, and you can lose 2 percent of your body weight in water. If it doesn't happen, be more wary of getting altitude illness; this doesn't mean that you will get altitude illness, just that you are more susceptible.

## Blood Response

At altitude the blood thickens, a process that takes a month or more to complete. Actually, in the first few days your blood gets thicker because of the diuresis and associated fluid loss. Later it gets thicker because the body makes more red blood cells to carry the oxygen. Using the freight train analogy again, if each train adds more boxcars (red blood cells), then it can carry more oxygen. This can be a problem if there are too many boxcars, each carrying a small payload. The train is too heavy and can't travel as fast or as efficiently; that is, your blood becomes too thick.

The blood of Sherpas who live at altitude does not thicken as much as that of lowlanders. Thick blood can clot easier, or can sludge and cause problems in delivering oxygen where it is needed. Inactivity, such as being confined in a tent by a storm for a few days, can increase the risk of developing a clot that could migrate. For example, blood clots in the legs can migrate to the lungs and cause life-threatening illness. Migrating clots may be a more common problem than previously thought and could explain the sudden rapid deterioration of people high up in the mountains. If caught in such a situation, force yourself to exercise. Go outside if possible. If you can't get out, do isometrics, or undertake make-work projects.

Some people have suggested that one should thin the blood by removing some of the extra red blood cells, but this doesn't appear to work. Others suggest that you take a drug such as aspirin, which will make the blood less sticky and less likely to clot. There are no studies of this at altitude. In some cases, thinning the blood could result in problems, such as increased bleeding from an injury or a stomach ulcer. Opinions on whether people should take aspirin at altitude are divided; it may make sense at extreme altitudes (above 18,000 ft. or 5,500 m) for those staying relatively long periods of time, but its effectiveness is not certain (most things aside from death and taxes are uncertain). I recommend aspirin for people who will spend more than a week at altitudes above 15,000 feet (4,500 m), especially if facing periods of inactivity. If you decide to take aspirin, one regular tablet (or even a baby aspirin tablet) every other day is adequate.

## Changes During Sleep

Most people at altitude do experience some difficulty getting to sleep. Sleep may be irregular, and some individuals may wake up breathless. This can happen at altitudes above 8,000 feet (2500 m), but is much more common sleeping at altitudes over 15,000 feet (4,500 m). In a tent, you may hear your companions' breathing increase and become loud, then decrease after a minute or two and become very quiet, almost imperceptible, or even cease, and then start up again. This pattern is called *periodic breathing*. Sometimes before breathing starts up again, the sleeper may awake, startled. This happens because during the initial phase of rapid breathing the body builds up oxygen in the brain, and the need to breathe diminishes. Just before the respiration becomes almost imperceptible, the brain, starved for oxygen, wakes the sleeper up to breathe! Periodic breathing often gives people anxiety and some may wish to abandon their trip. It is normal, however, and diminishes with acclimatization. Sleeping pills will make you breathe less, and as a result, less oxygen is delivered to the tissues—not a desirable state of affairs. Don't take sleeping pills, sedatives, or most tranquilizers, all of which have the same effect. Better ways to improve the quality of sleep are described later.

## High Altitude Deterioration

People don't live permanently above 16,500 feet (5,000 m) or so, for good reason: the body doesn't adapt well. The longer you stay at altitudes above 16,500 feet, the more you deteriorate physically, mentally, and emotionally. Some altitude researchers believe there is long-standing brain damage that occurs after staying above 16,500 feet for extended periods of time. There are plenty of climbers from the 1920s expeditions to Everest that went to altitudes of 28,000 feet (8,500 m) without oxygen, stayed at extreme altitude for considerable periods of time, and who then led productive intellectual lives. I wouldn't suggest you make your decision to avoid altitude activities because of the fear of brain damage.

## Optimum Period for Acclimatization

What is the best way for an individual to acclimatize? There is no hard and fast formula; it varies with each person for every exposure. A conservative estimate would be to increase the sleeping altitude by 1,000 feet (300 m) a night above 10,000 feet (3,050 m). While ascending, take a break every two to three days by sleeping at the same altitude as the previous day. You can also average the process and ascend 750 feet (230 m) a day. To make an alpine style ascent of an 8,000-meter (26,250-ft.) mountain, three weeks spent at altitudes around 19,685 feet (6,000

m) might be enough, although for some, it might be too short a period and for others, too long. For a 6,000-meter (19,685-ft.) trekking peak, seven to ten days of acclimatizing seems reasonable.

For those making journeys to intermediate altitudes, plan to arrive a day or two early, and take it easy at first. If you will be sleeping at an altitude of 10,000 feet (3,050 m) or so, sleep at an intermediate altitude the day before instead of making an abrupt ascent from your base elevation. Those coming from sea level to ski in Colorado or Utah might consider spending the night in Denver. Follow the rule of climb high but sleep low—meaning climb as high as you can during the day, but descend and sleep at the same elevation or a little higher than the night before. If you are not feeling well, don't raise your sleeping altitude at all. Exertion should be done to moderation; don't overexert.

In the final analysis, trial and error is the best way to discover the pace at which you, as an individual, need to acclimatize.

# Chapter 2. What is Altitude Illness?

It is helpful to define the terms *disease* (the opposite of ease, or lack of ease), *syndrome* and *illness,* based on the biomedical model. Disease, as used here, describes entities that are disorders of physiological or psychological function. An example of a disease is the common cold, which results from an infection by one of a group of cold viruses. A cold characteristically produces a runny nose, cough, sore throat, and so forth in its victims. As of yet there are no commonly agreed upon diseases of altitude that we understand in the same detail as the common cold.

By contrast, *illness* can be defined as a state in which an individual feels unwell. By this definition, *altitude illness* comprises all the problems associated with not feeling well at altitude.

The term *syndrome* refers to an association of *symptoms* (what the patient feels or complains about) and *signs* (what the health care practitioner sees, feels, listens to, or measures) that occur together more often than would be expected by chance. AIDS, standing for Acquired Immune Deficiency Syndrome, was originally used to describe such a group of symptoms or signs. AIDS is now recognized as an end point on a spectrum of disease caused by infection with the HIV virus. All of the illnesses of altitude—acute mountain sickness (AMS), high altitude pulmonary edema (HAPE), and high altitude cerebral edema (HACE), among others—are considered syndromes today. Are all of the altitude illnesses really one disease with different manifestations, such as HIV infection, or are they different? Eventually, they may all represent one disease, like symptomatic HIV infection.

*Sickness* can be defined as a role society bestows upon an individual. This individual's behavior is characterized by some deficit in physical or mental function. Calling acute mountain sickness (AMS) a sickness means that altitude savants (the society in question) have grouped people with certain symptoms and signs together, thinking these people may exhibit facets of a single disease that is not yet well understood. The answer to this question is unknown at present.

The point at which you feel the altitude (meaning that you sense a difference in functioning because of the altitude) varies with the speed of ascent and with your individual condition on a particular journey. Some people will feel the altitude at 6,000 feet (1,800 m); while most will feel it by 10,000 feet (3,050 m); and all will by 15,000 feet (4,575 m). Serious altitude illness such as HAPE or HACE can occur at altitudes around 10,000 feet (3,050 m), or even lower in some people, but are more common at higher altitudes. The likelihood of HAPE or HACE occurring will depend on how fast you ascend, your past history of adapting to altitude, and other factors that are less well understood.

It may be useful to consider altitude illness that occurs up to say, 18,000 feet (5,500 m) as altitude illness of acclimatization. Above this, altitude illness occurs as a part of a stay at extreme altitude where the physiology may be somewhat different than at more modest elevations. Higher, anything goes. It is much harder to study sick individuals above 18,000 feet, and our knowledge, for the most part, is based on reports rather than firsthand observation.

The syndromes of altitude illness will be described with the most common first. In the glossary, you'll find the clinical definitions agreed upon at the Hypoxia meetings in 1991 at Lake Louise.

## Acute Mountain Sickness (AMS)

*Acute Mountain Sickness* (AMS) is the most common form of altitude illness. In its mild form, it feels like a hangover. AMS often occurs around 8,000 feet (2,450 m) or higher but can occur at even lower altitudes. The most common symptom is a headache that responds to simple pain medicine, such as aspirin, acetaminophen (paracetamol), or ibuprofen. In addition, at least one of the following symptoms is present: nausea, lack of appetite, sleeplessness, or malaise (not feeling well in a vague way and not having much energy). AMS comes on one to three days after arrival at altitude and lasts about the same time, especially if the sleeping altitude is not raised. Although not serious by itself, it can progress to the more ominous moderate form. I make the distinctions between mild and moderate AMS to enable you to vigilantly look out for severe AMS. When experiencing the moderate form of altitude sickness, the victim usually vomits a time or two, has a headache that cannot be relieved by the usual pain medicines, and he or she can be very short of breath during mild exertion. After mild or moderate AMS resolves, further ascent is possible.

Severe AMS can be life threatening. It is characterized by altered balance and muscular coordination (called *ataxia* by the cognoscenti and those clinically inclined). This is the hallmark of severe AMS and may represent the earliest stage of its progression or potential progression to cerebral edema. Measure it by the tandem walking test, also called the drunk test or the state trooper test (see Chapter 4, section III). The victim may fumble, show poor coordination, and experience an *altered mental state* in which he or she is not thinking clearly and seems unaware of surroundings and external events. Such a person may be angry, combative, or incomprehensible. Sometimes, extreme shortness of breath with almost any activity can be observed. After severe AMS, further ascent is not advised unless there are options for easy and rapid descent should symptoms recur.

If there are no other symptoms, it may be difficult to distinguish severe AMS from fatigue, stress, and dehydration. Also, conditions such as heat illness, exhaustion, infections such as sinusitis or malaria, and carbon monoxide poisoning from cooking inside a snow-covered tent or snow cave may also be the cause.

Individuals at greater risk of AMS are: those who make a rapid ascent, especially using a car, train or plane for part of their journey and who thus raise their sleeping altitude abruptly; those who have had AMS before; and those who gain weight or retain fluid at altitude or who do not urinate excessively after arrival. Obesity and lung disease are probable risk factors as is residence at sea level compared to residence at 5,000 feet (1,500 m) or higher.

## High Altitude Pulmonary Edema (HAPE)

*High Altitude Pulmonary Edema* (HAPE) results from an accumulation of fluid that comes from the blood and leaks into the oxygen-exchanging air sacs of the lungs. Lack of oxygen in the air coupled with high pressure in the arteries supplying the lungs promote this condition, and it is exacerbated by cold, exercise, and dehydration. HAPE may affect one or two percent of those going up high and commonly occurs on the second night after arrival at altitude.

The HAPE victim may awake from sleep with extreme difficulty breathing. Unlike an individual experiencing periodic breathing, a person suffering from HAPE will not be able to catch his breath and will find it very difficult to exert himself to any extent. During the day, the earliest symptom experienced may be slightly decreased exercise performance, but by itself, this is usually not a helpful observation. The victim's breathing will be fast (more than thirty times a minute in severe cases), and he or she will experience severe breathlessness at rest and will be unable to catch his or her breath or speak in full sentences. In some cases, individuals with HAPE complain only of weakness. Most people who get HAPE will already be suffering from AMS. HAPE may be more common among those exercising more, such as extreme climbers, than among less active trekkers.

As HAPE gets worse, the victim becomes incapable of any significant physical exertion or activity. The pulse is rapid, so that if a person has been monitoring his resting pulse at altitude, he will notice a considerable increase. In more severe cases, there will be a cough, often dry, though bubbly or productive (that is, producing considerable sputum). Fever is often present; for years doctors diagnosed this condition as pneumonia that failed to respond to antibiotics. As HAPE gets worse, the victim's color will be bluer than that of his companions (compare the color of lips or fingernail beds in daylight), reflecting his or her lungs' inability to transport oxygen into the blood. This is termed *cyanosis*. In rare circumstances HAPE may be accompanied by HACE. Those who are experienced in listening to the lungs may hear rales (crackles) when pressing the ear tightly against the chest wall; a stethoscope isn't necessary. They may be detected first by listening at the level of the right nipple, below the armpit. Hearing these sounds by themselves, in the absence of other symptoms, is not helpful, as many people have rales at altitude. Rales should not be present in the normal person after several deep breaths. Individuals can also complain of chest tightness or congestion. HAPE rarely occurs at altitudes below 8,000 feet (2,450 m). Children seem to be more susceptible. Young adult males are also thought to be more susceptible, but this may appear so because they expose themselves more to the risks of the syndrome.

HAPE can affect residents of high altitudes when they return to high altitude after descending to an elevation below 8,000 feet (2,450 m). It is more likely to affect both males and females below twenty years of age and is called re-entry or resident re-ascent HAPE.

Sometimes HAPE has been thought to occur after staying at altitude for a considerable time after which acclimatization should have occurred. Many of these people died without the true cause of death being determined. Blood clots migrating from the legs to the lungs can be fatal. In addition, a hole in the heart, normally present only during fetal growth, might open at altitude (termed a patent foramen ovale) and allow clots to pass to the brain, causing a rapid demise.

Current ideas suggest that the fluid in the air sacs results from a lung leak, rather than a lung injury. Thus if a person recovers quickly from this condition, is prudent about re-ascent, and takes medicine to prevent HAPE's recurrence, it may be possible to ascend again successfully.

HAPE is a serious condition, which can have a high fatality rate if untreated. Even if treated, some will still die, especially if appropriate treatment was begun late in the illness. Once HAPE comes on, it can rapidly progress to death. Recovery, however, is usually total with the only consequence being a predisposition to a recurrence of HAPE on revisiting high altitude destinations.

Risk factors for HAPE include prior HAPE, obesity, and the rare absence of a right pulmonary artery.

## High Altitude Cerebral Edema (HACE)

*High Altitude Cerebral Edema* (HACE), more rare than HAPE, is related to severe AMS. HACE is felt to be caused by swelling in the brain, as the organ gets waterlogged from dilation of its oxygen-starved blood vessels. The earliest sign of HACE is ataxia, or loss of balance and muscular coordination, as determined by the tandem walking test (see Chapter 4, section III). Ataxia or severe lassitude may remain the only sign for a period of time; coma may rapidly follow. An altered mental status or decreased mental functioning is usually present and will often progress, if untreated, to coma and death. Other symptoms can include hallucinations, weakness or numbness on one side of the body, being unable to talk, or being unable to make sense while talking. A headache is almost universal; nausea and vomiting are common. In addition, symptoms of HAPE may be present.

HACE is serious, with a high mortality rate if untreated, and has occurred at altitudes as low as 10,000 feet (3,050 m). Symptoms usually clear quickly with descent but sometimes can persist for days. Those who recover rarely can have evidence of permanent neurological injury. Some experts ascribe this damage to other conditions.

## High Altitude Edema

*High altitude edema* or swelling of the hands, face, and ankles is common, affecting perhaps one in five of those trekking to 14,000 feet (4,275 m). Twice as common in women than in men it is also more frequent in those with AMS. Not serious by itself, it should alert the victim and others to look at other more perilous forms of altitude illness, including severe AMS and HAPE.

## High Altitude Retinopathy

*High altitude retinopathy* refers to changes in the retina of the eye: bleeding and other pathology. Usually this is not apparent to the person or companions, unless the changes occur in the macula, a part of the retina where the eyesight is most sensitive. In this case, the person will notice a loss of sharp vision. Retinopathy is common in people going above 15,000 feet (4,575 m) and is almost universal above 26,250 feet (8,000 m). The condition clears with descent.

## High Altitude Syncope

*Syncope,* a medical term denoting a brief loss of consciousness, is called "fainting" by lay people. In some cases, people who have arrived at 8,200 to 10,000 feet (2,500 to 3,000 m) the previous day stand up after eating and faint. They recover quickly, however, without further problems. Whether *high altitude syncope* really is an entity relating to altitude exposure is unclear. Other diseases may cause syncope and require medical attention. Making decisions on what to do in this circumstance is dependent on knowing more about the health of the individual who has fainted and requires considerable clinical judgment. The myriad causes of syncope are beyond the scope of this book.

## High Altitude Flatus Expulsion (HAFE)

HAFE, increased intestinal gas production at altitude, remains unstudied. Most flatulent people and their companions find it annoying. Some individuals alternate burps and farts with each step up. Swallowing extra air while gasping for breath may be a factor. HAFE does not result in serious harm.

Most of these syndromes can be prevented; see the next chapter.

# Chapter 3. Preventing Altitude Illness

Altitude illness can be avoided by ascending slowly and by raising the sleeping elevation gradually. How fast is slow enough is an individual phenomenon, and the rate that worked for an individual on one trip, may not work on the next. On some trips, you may acclimatize faster than on others. As suggested earlier, when traveling above 10,000 feet (3,050 m), try not to raise the sleeping altitude more than 1,000 feet (300 m) a day. This guideline may be too slow for some, and too fast for a few. A common strategy is to climb high during the day but descend to sleep at an altitude not more than a thousand feet above where you slept the night before. Don't overexert. For every three days above 10,000 feet (3,050 m), add an extra day at the previous night's sleeping altitude to the schedule. Arrange the itinerary to acclimatize slowly. Some people, no matter how hard they try, seem to hit a brick wall at a certain elevation and cannot go higher. When you take enough time to acclimatize, you lessen the risk of developing serious altitude illness and increase your performance and enjoyment in high altitude activities.

Mountaineers and climbers are risk takers of a different sort than the more casual skier, hiker, or trekker. The fatality rate on the highest Himalayan climbs approaches 3 percent, apparently an acceptable "risk factory" to a subset of the mountaineering population. Some exhibit a "do or die" mentality and consider altitude illness an occupational hazard. They may not heed the cautions about slow ascent in this book and may be eager to try pharmacotherapy to help achieve summits. The great Himalayan climbers are very conscious about acclimatization and listen to an inner sense, based on experience, to determine when they are ready to go higher.

Climbers and others going to high altitudes may wish to "pre-acclimatize" themselves in a hypobaric chamber. Some experts have advocated spending time in such a device, usually found in research military bases, but few will have these resources. Currently, a type of high altitude bed, also known as a High Altitude Training Chamber (HATCH) or hypobaric bag, is now available. In a high altitude bed, the principle of climbing high and sleeping low is reversed: the individual sleeps high and trains low to get the advantages of blood doping in a holistic fashion, making the blood thicker so it has more oxygen-carrying capacity. Prototypes have been used by climbers before departing for 8,000-meter peak climbs. The source is listed in Chapter 5 under Hyperbaric Chamber (Gamow Bag®).

It is preferable, however, to use a natural "chamber" by going to an altitude destination a week or so before departure for a higher one. Spend as long as you can in the natural "chamber" to benefit from the residual acclimatization effect, which lasts a few days to a week or two and depends on the individual as well as the altitude of the "chamber."

Those contemplating an alpine style ascent of a major mountain usually can't follow the ascent strategy recommended earlier. In that case, spend considerable time acclimatizing at the base camp and make daily ascents to monitor the effectiveness of your performance at altitude. You will have a sense of when you are ready to push up.

Keep drinking. Does hydrating prevent altitude illness? By itself, probably not, but increasing your water intake is a vital factor in promoting well being. The altitude environment is usually a dry one, and living and exercising there promotes increased water loss. If you take a diuretic such as acetazolamide (mentioned below) to prevent altitude illness, you will urinate more and water loss will be increased. Therefore, drinking more fluids is necessary. Recommending that you increase your water intake to prevent altitude illness may seem paradoxical when the syndromes of altitude illness appear to result from too much water in the brain and lungs. But the fact is, you need enough fluid in your circulatory system to keep it functioning well. One recommendation is to drink sufficient water to produce two bursting bladders full of urine a day. If your urine has a strong yellow concentrated color, you're not drinking enough. The mustard-colored snow surrounding expedition tents on high mountain climbs attests to the difficulties of following this advice. People may not perceive their own bladder capacity accurately, so many experienced trip leaders recommend drinking at least four quarts (liters) of fluid a day. Drinking enough is easier if your water bottle is accessible and insulated, if in extreme cold. At moderate altitudes, drink a couple of quarts (liters) a day.

Keeping warm helps lessen the rise of pulmonary artery pressures in the lungs and decreases the risk of HAPE. Temperature falls as you gain altitude. Dehydration, cold, and the lack of oxygen at altitude are synergistic in producing HAPE. Individuals who leave warm sea-level climates may not bring clothing adequate for travel at high altitudes. Minimizing the number of times you need to stop and adjust clothing during the day will decrease fatigue. If possible, anticipate clothing changes and take off a jacket before you climb uphill, or put on insulation as soon as you stop, before you cool down. Choose clothing items that allow variable ventilation and permit adjustment and removal while moving. Garments with side and underarm zippers that allow the arms to be removed entirely from the sleeves while exercising are optimal. Being able to dress appropriately for high altitude situations comes with experience, from observing others, and from discussions with veterans.

Diet is important. Eat enough food, whatever is palatable, and avoid excesses of salt. If you have a good appetite up high it is unlikely that you have significant altitude illness. Pass up alcoholic beverages, at least until you are acclimatized.

Mild exercise can enhance altitude adaptation but strenuous activity could promote HAPE. Motivated athletes, used to exercising to exhaustion, may attempt this level of exertion up high and push beyond where normal individuals might stop. A better tactic is to increase the activity level gradually, and take it easy the first few days up high. Newcomers to the heights are usually surprised at how much more slowly they function; vigorous activity before they acclimatize is usually out of the question. Fatigue will increase at altitude, so adjust the pace to insure that you will have enough strength to finish the activity with some left for contingencies. Since a major part of adapting to altitude involves breathing more, many climbers feel consciously doing so helps.

Acetazolamide can be useful in preventing altitude illness, especially AMS, and is FDA approved for this purpose. Taking this drug makes physiologic sense as it allows you to breathe more and speeds acclimatization. Acetazolamide helps the body excrete bicarbonate produced from carbon dioxide, a product of metabolism. In our freight train analogy, it makes the loader work faster. It is recommended for those flying or driving to altitude on tight schedules, or for climbers having to raise their sleeping altitude by 2,000 feet (610 m) or more a day when above 10,000 feet (3,050 m). Individuals who have had altitude illness on previous occasions may be helped by it. I do not recommend it for the average individual traveling from near sea level to altitude in the U.S. mountain states for a brief ski vacation.

The dose is 125 mg (break a 250 mg tablet in half) twice a day. Although lower than the previously recommended dose, 125 mg is as effective as the higher doses, produces less water loss through urination than 250 mg, and causes fewer side effects. You can stop taking it after one or two days at the same altitude. Commonly reported side effects are tingling of the fingers, toes, and the area around the lips, frequent urination (it acts as a diuretic), and having the perception that carbonated beverages taste flat. Acetazolamide is a sulfa drug and should not be taken by those allergic to sulfas. There are no data on its use for children. You could try a dose of 2–5 mg/kg twice a day.

Another drug that prevents altitude illness is dexamethasone, a potent corticosteroid. Because of steroidal side effects, the possibility of rebound altitude illness when it is stopped, and the fact that it doesn't aid acclimatization, it is only recommended for those who have to land at high altitude by aircraft to do rescue work; then it should be taken with acetazolamide. People allergic to sulfa drugs who need to take a drug for prophylaxis might consider it. The dose is four mg every six hours. Don't take it for more than five days. Many people report feeling bad while taking it or after stopping it; others experience euphoria. One climber reported feeling weak, lethargic, and depressed for a month after taking dexamethasone. Azetazolamide and dexamethasone may work better together than either separately.

Travelers who have had HAPE before and wish to go to altitude can take nifedipine to lessen the chances of recurrence. Nifedipine dilates the pulmonary arteries; in our metaphor, it widens the roadway of the loader. The recommended dose is 20 mg of the slow-release preparation every six hours or 30 to 60 mg of the 30 mg extended tablet once a day. Since a nifedipine can signficantly lower blood pressure, it is best to have your doctor instruct you in how to use this potentially hazardous drug. Slow ascent is still the most important advice in HAPE prevention.

Behavioral characteristics may be important in preventing altitude illness. Goal-oriented and driven people may be more at risk, as they will push themselves to go higher and deny symptoms of altitude illness. People traveling independently tend to stop and rest for a day when they feel ill. Those on adventure travel group trips, in contrast, may be more likely to die from altitude illness; this observation is based on data from Nepal (see Shlim, 1992). Such groups, if not carefully planned and guided, tend to stick to a fixed schedule. A preestablished itinerary may be too fast to allow certain individuals to acclimatize, making them more vulnerable to altitude illness. Peer pressure may push someone to ascend faster than he or she otherwise would. It also makes it difficult for an individual to admit having symptoms for fear of slowing down the group or of being left behind. Since splitting a party to accommodate a slow acclimatizer might pose logistical problems, the leader may hesitate diagnosing altitude illness. See Evaluating Modes of Travel at Altitude in Chapter 7 to learn how to evaluate a commercial operator.

Competitive athletes may combine living at altitude with training near sea level to improve sea level performance. Exercise performance at altitude may also be enhanced by this philosophy. Optimal living altitudes of 8200–9200 ft (2500–2800 m) combined with high intensity interval workouts below 5000 ft (1500 m) may produce the greatest performance improvement for low altitude events. See Levine (1995) for an exercise physiologist's perspective.

## Maximizing Your Enjoyment at Altitude

- Raise your sleeping altitude by no more that 1,000 ft. (305 m) each night above 10,000 ft. (3050 M).
- Climb as high as you like each day as long as you follow the "sleeping altitude" rule.
- Build in a sleeping-altitude halt every 3,000 ft. (1,000 m).
- Spend at least one night below 10,000 ft (3050 m) before ascending higher.

- If you don't feel good, do not raise your sleeping altitude until you feel better.
- If you don't get better by staying at your current sleeping altitude, go down to below where you first felt sick.
- Don't take a headache higher under any circumstances.
- Be especially concerned and vigilant if a headache comes on during the day's ascent and gets worse.
- Don't urinate into the wind, or uphill if there is any wind.

On your trip you will encounter altitude illness. Determining which type and what to do is covered next.

# Chapter 4. Diagnosing Altitude Illness

An illness at altitude is altitude illness until *proven* otherwise. Victims often ascribe symptoms of altitude illness to a flu-like condition, sinusitis, dehydration, pneumonia, bronchitis, a hangover, or an ear infection, which can all present with similar symptoms. The most likely cause up high, however, is altitude illness. They commonly deny that they are suffering from altitude illness because they don't want to face the effect this has on ego, self-image, and their relationships with others in the group. Altitude illness is a legitimate affliction. It is not a sign of weak character or lack of conditioning.

Section I describes a systematic approach to diagnose and treat altitude illness. Like a botanical key or a decision tree, choose among pairs of statements to get to the presumptive diagnosis and treatment you need. The protocol, properly followed, should direct you to adequately treat ninety percent or more of the cases of serious altitude illness. Take notes as you go through the list. The next chapter details these treatments.

In Section II, you'll find a simpler approach to making a decision about ascending or descending. An alternative approach to these algorithms in Section IV compares your functioning with that of your companions and to some objective parameters. In your travel it is not slowness per se at issue. Guides report that some of their best clients are those with the wisdom to move at their own pace, which may be slow but steady. The harbinger of altitude illness is non-recovery from tiredness or exhaustion, whatever the pace.

At altitude, the lack of oxygen may affect the examiner's judgment as well. If possible, involve several people who don't appear to have altitude illness in the evaluation to arrive at a better decision.

## I. A Systematic Approach to Diagnose and Treat Altitude Illness

*If the suspected victim of altitude illness is not doing well or having complaints,* go through the following list from No. 1 to No. 10 sequentially. If the person is in a coma (is unconscious), go to No. 6.

1. **Are the ascent profile, signs, and symptoms compatible with altitude illness?** Talk to the suspected victim or companions about what he did on which days, how he performed doing those activities, at what altitude he slept, and how he felt. From his or her answers, you should be able to determine whether or not the problem is due to altitude, and if so, what is the probable altitude syndrome the victim has. If the person has been well and has descended a high pass, returned to a lower altitude, then develops, say, fevers, shaking, chills, and a cough, HAPE is unlikely. In a simple ski or mountain ascent, the profile is obvious, but on a Himalayan trek across several high passes or an expeditionary climb with many carries to stock high camps, there will be many variations to the altitude profile. Altitude illness rarely has a dramatic presentation, it begins insidiously and progresses. You won't see cases where an individual feels strong and energetic enough to complete a difficult ice pitch at altitude, and then suddenly collapses with serious altitude illness.

    A. *If no,* treat the most likely cause. Descent will probably be an important part of that treatment if the condition is serious.

    B. *If yes,* evaluate the following:

2. **Is there a headache?**

    A. *If yes,* follow Dr. Peter Hackett's headache rule: Rest, do not ascend further, snack, drink fluids, and take mild pain medicine.

        i. *If better and there are no other symptoms,* continue with the activity.

        ii. *If better and there are other symptoms,* see No. 3 to No. 10. Check for ataxia below.

        iii. *If not better,* then:

            a. *Test for **ataxia**,* using the tandem walking test. (See section III.)

                • *If yes,* take the person down immediately (read descent in the next chapter) and give dexamethasone and oxygen. The hyperbaric bag can be a temporizing step if available.

- *If negative,* rest at that altitude and test again for ataxia in six to twelve hours.

B. *Test for **altered mental status*** by asking the person to do simple arithmetic, such as subtracting 7 sequentially from 99 (answer is 92, 85, 78, 71, 64, etc.), or ask if he or she is aware of current events, specific dates, and so forth.

   i. *If there is altered mental status*

      a. *Check for state of **hydration.*** If in doubt as to whether severe dehydration is the cause, rehydrate, have the person descend, and re-evaluate. Be certain the individual is not **hypothermic** (cold) and suffering from exposure, in which case rewarming is necessary. One way to check the state of hydration is to measure the pulse with the person lying down, then have him or her stand up, wait 1–2 minutes and note the rise. If it goes up by twenty-five beats per minute, it suggests that significant dehydration is present. Or ask about or look at the urine color (strong yellow implies dehydration) and examine the lips and mouth to see how dry they appear.

   ii. *If altered mental status is not present,* retest for ataxia and mental status changes in twelve hours.

C. *If no headache,* check 2. A. iii and the following:

**3. Is the person short of breath?**

A. *If yes,* let the victim rest for fifteen minutes and see if he or she recovers.

   i. *If the victim doesn't recover,* limit further exertion, and treat for HAPE by descent with limited exertion. Give oxygen if available

      a. *If descent is not possible,* have the victim rest.

- Give a trial of the hyperbaric bag, or oxygen if available.
- If oxygen or a hyperbaric bag are not available, give nifedipine. (See Drugs in Chapter 5 for the protocol to use with this drug.)

      ii. *If the victim recovers from shortness of breath* in fifteen minutes and there are no other symptoms, continue with the activity.

   B. If the victim is not short of breath, check the following:

**4.   Does the person have a good appetite?**

   A. *If yes,* then significant altitude illness is probably not present but check No. 5 to No. 10.

   B. *If no,* and the person has not been urinating copiously and there are none of the other symptoms or signs described above, besides a mild headache, return to the previous night's sleeping altitude to sleep and rest for a day. Re-evaluate in twelve hours.

   C. *If no,* and the person has been urinating copiously, continue with the activity and re-evaluate in twelve hours.

**5.   Is person experiencing severely blurred or decreased vision?**

   A. *If yes,* then give the victim oxygen and/or hyperbaric therapy, and descend.

   B. *If no,* check the following:

**6.   Did the person faint?**

   A. *If the person is in a coma,* treat for HACE and give dexamethasone by injection, as well as the usual first aid measures for a comatose victim. ***Descend as soon as possible and evacuate***.

   B. *If yes,* ask about other health problems the person has had.

      i. If there are other causes treat the likely ones appropriately.

      ii. If there are no other causes, did he or she recover quickly (in a matter of minutes)?

         a. *If no,* give oxygen or hyperbaric therapy, and descend.

         b. *If yes,* check for other symptoms of altitude illness and treat accordingly. Do not sleep any higher than the night before.

   C. *If no fainting has occurred,* check the following:

**7.   Does the person have swelling of the face, hands, or feet?**

   A. *If yes,* check for the other symptoms in this list.

      i. *If other symptoms are present,* treat those and re-evaluate in twelve hours.

      ii. *If no other symptoms are present,* recheck in twelve to twenty-four hours.

      iii. *If the swelling is extremely uncomfortable* and a diuretic such as furosemide is available, administer as described below. (See Drugs in Chapter 5.)

    B. *If no,* then serious altitude illness is probably not present, given that no other symptoms listed above exist.

**8. Is the person experiencing difficulty sleeping?**

    A. *If yes,* ask companions if periodic breathing is present.

      i. *If yes or unsure,* then give the person acetazolamide 125 mg at bedtime for three to four days; do not give sleeping pills.

      ii. *If no,* treat the companions for difficulty sleeping!

    B. *If no,* reassure the person, advise against taking sleeping pills and check the following.

**9. Is the person anxious, disoriented, irritable, or more emotional?**

    A. *If yes,* go back to No. 2 and re-test for ataxia and altered mental status and follow that protocol.

    B. *If no,* go on to No. 10.

**10. Get answers to the following questions:**

    A. Has the person had altitude problems before?

      i. At what altitude, which symptoms, and what was done about it? Use this information to guide further treatment (a favorite method used by astute clinicians to treat difficult cases).

    B. Does the person have other health problems? Oftentimes the person will have preexisting health problems that may be the cause of his or her discomfort. If doubtful, descent is the best recourse.

    C. What does the victim think is going on? (Ask companions this too, it will make you a wise clinician.) Consider the answers you get in making decisions.

      D. Is the person consuming mood-altering drugs, including al-
         cohol?
         i. If yes, stop consuming those. Be prepared to deal with
           withdrawal symptoms. Descent may be in order.

### *Monitoring Altitude Illness*

To gauge the response to your treatment, measure and record the heart
and respiratory rates, listing them together with the symptoms and signs,
noting observation times. Repeat the assessment frequently, say at inter-
vals of four to twenty-four hours depending on the severity of the illness.

## II. Simplified Decision Tree

Begin by following No.1 in Section I above to see if the symptoms
and signs are compatible with altitude illness.
      A. If altitude illness is suspected, don't ascend.
      B. Descend if you don't get better, or immediately if:
         1. there is severe shortness of breath at rest; that is, the
           victim doesn't catch his or her breath after resting 15
           minutes.
         2. ataxia is present.
         3. there is no improvement in the symptoms and signs
           while resting at the same altitude.
         4. the person is getting worse.
         5. confusion or hallucinations are present.
      C. If you ascend with altitude illness, you will get worse.

## III. Tests to Demonstrate Ataxia

Let the subject who is having difficulty at altitude rest. Then administer the **tandem walking test.** Draw a straight line at least 6 feet (2 m)
long on the ground or in the snow with the heel of a boot or a stick.
Choose a safe level place with no rocks or debris. Demonstrate how to
walk along the line, putting the heel of the foot ahead touching the toe
of the foot behind. Have the subject attempt this. Slight difficulty, using
the arms for balance, is tolerable if 12 feet (4 m.) can be covered in a
straight line. If the person steps off the line or falls to the ground, the
test is abnormal. Assuming you do not have severe AMS yourself, your

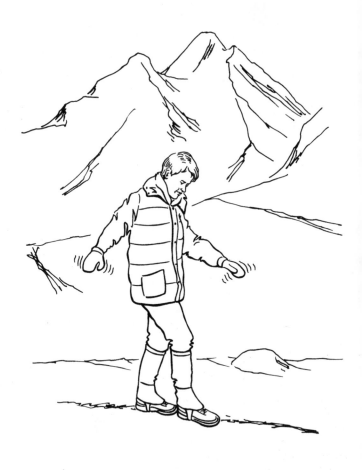

*Tandem walking test*

competence in doing this serves as a control to assess the potential victim. Rugged terrain may make it more difficult for both of you to accomplish the maneuver. With exhaustion, hypothermia, or mild intoxication, some loss of coordination (ataxia) can be seen, but there should be no staggering or falling. Another test is to have the person stand, feet together, arms at the side (or held out in front), and eyes closed. If the person sways considerably, significant loss of coordination (ataxia) is present, but this is not as sensitive as the tandem walking test. Again, use an unaffected member of the party as a measure.

## IV. Altitude Illness in Yourself and Your Companions

*Symptoms or signs to look for **in yourself*** that would lead you to suspect significant altitude illness:

A. Resting pulse above 110 per minute.
 1. Be especially wary if your pulse at altitude goes up after having been at altitude for a while.
 2. Measure your pulse in the same circumstance each time, say lying in a tent in the morning.
 3. Your pulse may go up from caffeine or anxiety, but should not remain high after resting.
B. If you are on certain medicines used to control the heart beat or blood pressure, treat angina or prevent migraine headaches (see Pulse Increase in Chapter 1) you may not have a high resting pulse and yet still have altitude illness.
C. Marked shortness of breath at rest (after you have recovered from the activity and are breathing more than twenty times a minute).
D. Loss of appetite.
E. Great fatigue while undertaking an activity, especially if it is increasing in comparison to your companions' level of fatigue.

*Signs to look for **in your companions*** suggesting significant altitude illness:

A. Someone skipping meals and wanting to spend more time in the tent

B. Changes in behavior. For example, someone who:
   1. becomes quiet and retiring when he or she had been gregarious before.
   2. is a quiet person becomes quieter.
   3. becomes obnoxious. You notice new difficulties in getting along with this person.
   4. is persistently very somnolent.
C. An individual having more trouble with an activity than his or her companions, especially if this is not the case usually. For example:
   1. if trekking, this person is the most tired on arrival at the destination.
   2. if skiing, this person is constantly falling and is the slowest.
   3. if climbing, this person is getting much slower and is less competent when doing technical climbing.
   4. if during a group meeting, this person becomes forgetful and loses the theme of the discussion.

The following are the best ways to confirm the suspicion of altitude illness if the signs and symptoms described above are present.

A. Increase the victim's oxygen intake either by 1) having the victim descend, 2) giving oxygen by mask or 3) placing the victim in a hyperbaric bag and observing the response. Descent is the preferred option.
B. Wait at a specific altitude that is no higher than the previous night's sleeping altitude and see if the victim gets better. This is only recommended for those who have mild to moderate AMS, or high altitude edema, not for High Altitude *Pulmonary* Edema (HAPE) when immediate descent is necessary.

Details on the treatment options follow.

# Diagnosing Altitude Illness in Children

In young children diagnosing altitude illness is difficult, especially since the parents may not be such astute observers as they are at lower altitudes. If the child's color is blue or dusky, go down. If the child is not playing, becomes fussy, is not eating, or is very sleepy, and if you as parents are more concerned with how you are adapting to the altitude, or are focussed on the views at altitude and are neglecting your children, go down.

# Chapter 5. Treatment of Altitude Illness

Various methods for treating altitude illness for the non-medical practitioner are described in this chapter. Treatment for severe AMS and for presumed HAPE and HACE are given together. Treatment protocols for health care providers in a clinical facility at intermediate altitude are outlined separately.

## Descent

Altitude guru Dr. Peter Hackett said some time ago that there were three rules for treating altitude illness: descent, descent, descent! This remains the gold standard of care. It is never a poor decision.

These days, with other treatment modalities available, it is sometimes easy to forget the gold standard, and the consequences can be fatal! Descent is usually the most appropriate treatment. To see an improvement, it's usually necessary to descend 1,000 to 3,000 feet (300 to 1,000 m). Note the altitude at which even mild symptoms first occurred; that altitude becomes the individual's threshold of altitude illness on this occasion. Descend below that altitude after serious symptoms develop.

**Make every effort to get the victim down early, relying on his or her own ability to walk. Don't wait for the person to stagger or become unconscious and require evacuation.** If you take this advice to heart, you may need to insist on going down against the protestations of the sick person, who is determined to be "tough." Take charge, don't be polite.

When HAPE is suspected, minimize exertion. Have the victim transported if possible, by yak or on someone's back if there are no other vehicles. Self-descent in very early stages of HAPE is acceptable. Bad weather and hazardous terrain can stall the decision to evacuate to a lower altitude, a dire circumstance. Skilled mountaineering judgment regarding the safety of a descent must be weighed against the severity of the illness. Waiting for an air rescue can take several days in many situations, while altitude illness can progress to death in hours!

The first symptom to improve with descent is usually confusion and other alterations in mental status. The last to improve may be the loss of coordination, or ataxia.

# Oxygen

Oxygen, if available, should be given in all cases other than mild or moderate AMS. There is no harm in giving oxygen at altitude. Use a mask or nasal prongs for delivery at flows of two to four liters a minute in mild HAPE or early HACE. In more severe disease, a face mask and higher flows of eight to ten liters are necessary. When there is some response, decrease the dose to a level that is high enough to maintain the improvement. If there is no response, increase the dose to twelve liters per minute. Some noticeable response should occur in an hour, but sometimes it doesn't. Continue the oxygen and then consider other modes of treatment. Get the person down while giving oxygen.

On Denali (Mount McKinley), climbers on the West Buttress route with HAPE are given supplemental oxygen to breathe at 14,000 ft (4267 m), then they descend to 7,300 ft. (2,225 m) where they rest for 2–3 days before considering ascending again.

# Hyperbaric Chamber (Gamow Bag®)

Igor Gamow developed a portable fabric tube cylinder to accommodate a victim of altitude illness. Inflated by a foot pump to produce a pressure of 2 psi (103 mm Hg) over existing air pressure it simulates a descent of several thousand feet. Pump strokes every five seconds maintain the pressure. The higher the bag is used, the greater the relative descent. Groups going to altitudes above 15,000 feet (4,575 m) to trek or climb should consider purchasing or renting one. There are three versions, an Australian, a U.S. and a European one. Though expensive, the bag is cheaper than a coffin!

Advantages of the hyperbaric bag over oxygen stem from its compact size and low weight. As well, you cannot run out of air to pressurize it so it can be used over and over to re-treat the victim or to treat others. Oxygen is more bulky, heavier, and cylinders run out. Be sure to test the bag first before taking it along, because it can leak or the pump can malfunction. A Thermarest® patch applied to the inside can salvage a leaky bag. Compared to descent, once you use the bag and come out of it, you are still at the high altitude.

Someone with mild to moderate AMS might benefit from an hour or two in the bag, though this may not represent a significant improvement over just resting and using mild analgesics for twenty-four hours. Even if he or she gets better, the victim should be watched carefully to see if symptoms return. If symptoms are only mild, the person can stay at that altitude, but if more severe symptoms come on descent is appropriate.

If descent is not possible, those with severe symptoms of AMS or symptoms of HAPE or HACE should be treated in the bag for four to six hours. When anything other than mild HAPE is suspected, and if the person improves, he or she should subsequently descend and take medicines as outlined below. A victim treated with the bag should continue to have access to the bag until he or she is clearly better or has descended to below the point where the first symptoms of altitude illness occurred. Use the bag for the serious conditions when descent is impossible or too risky because of terrain, time, or weather. It may not work as well for HAPE as it does for HACE. Patients with severe HAPE can find it very uncomfortable to lie flat in the small models.

Before putting the victim into the bag, read the instructions that come with it. Attend to urination and defecation beforehand. Put a pee bottle in with the afflicted climber. Explain to the subject the need to breathe normally and to pop one's ears by swallowing or blowing gently against the pinched nose as the bag is inflated. Tell the victim that if the bag should suddenly deflate, he or she should exhale. Before closing the zipper, ask the subject to extend his arms and legs fully to increase the airspace inside the bag to save time and effort during inflation. Once inflated, about ten to twenty pumps a minute are usually necessary.

When the bag is used, an observer should be with the victim at all times. If the person vomits, get him out of the bag immediately and clear the airway. A drowsy climber with decreased mental function can inhale the vomitus. Considerable effort is needed to keep a person in the bag to maintain the pressure. While it may save lives by buying time, using the bag ordinarily only postpones the need to descend. When using a hyperbaric bag, the victim may feel claustrophobic and may also have difficulties clearing the ears and sinuses as pressure increases. In one case, an individual with severe altitude illness used the bag, improved, tried to avoid descent, and subsequently died when the bag was no longer available to re-treat recurrent altitude illness.

The current models use a dry-suit zipper as a seal. The zipper's durability may limit the number of seasons a bag can remain functional. Valves are prone to breakdown as well.

The sources for the three currently available models are:

Chinook Medical Gear, P.O, Box 1736, Edwards, CO 81632, (800) 766-1365, (970) 926-9277, Fax (970) 926-9660, chinook@vail.net, http://www.chinookmed.com for the Gamow Bag and the High Altitude Training Chamber, as well as for other travel health and altitude illness treatment supplies.

Certec, le bourge, Sourcieux le Mines, 69210 L'Arbresle, France, 33-74-70-3982, Fax 33-74-70-3766, probably the strongest version.

C.E. Bartlett Pty Ltd. Ring Road, Wendouree, Victoria 3355, Australia, (61) 3 5339 3101, Fax (61) 3 5338 1241, info@bartlett.net.au, http://www.bartlett.net.au for the PAC (Portable Altitude Chamber), currently the cheapest version and the easiest to get patients in and out of.

# Drugs

### ACETAZOLAMIDE

Acetazolamide is recommended for treating symptoms of AMS of any degree in adults. Although unlikely to make a great difference in severe AMS, it should be taken nevertheless. To simply improve sleep, the dose for mild AMS can be as low as 125 mg, taken at bedtime. For moderate to severe AMS, increase it to 250 mg twice a day which can be continued until the victim feels much better. Common side effects include increased urination, numbness or tingling of the hands, feet, and the area around the mouth, nausea, and having carbonated beverages taste flat. Some individuals find these side effects unacceptable and cannot tolerate this drug. Since it is a sulfa drug, it should not be taken by those allergic to sulfas. While it is safe to give to children, there is no experience in using it at altitude with this population.

For mild to moderate AMS, acetazolamide coupled with not raising the sleeping altitude may be sufficient treatment. In all other situations, it is an adjunct. Other treatments are required.

## NIFEDIPINE

For a victim suffering from mild HAPE (the person is capable of some physical activity) and no other altitude illness other than mild AMS, giving nifedipine may effectively treat the condition. He or she may be able to stay at altitude until improved and then descend or possibly ascend (see below). In more severe cases, urgent descent and other treatment in addition to nifedipine will be necessary. Monitor the dose and the response and use judgment to adjust the dose where necessary.

Rarely, treatment with nifedipine can lower blood pressure enough to cause someone to fall or faint. (Once, it prevented a climber from standing up in a precarious position. Even more disastrous situations can be imagined.) When using this drug, avoid being in a potentially hazardous situation and have a responsible individual monitor the response. Only give nifedipine and undertake descent if the victim is being carried or otherwise conveyed. Fortunately, the problem of fainting or having a serious drop in blood pressure when taking nifedipine has not occurred often at altitude.

Performing a nifedipine treatment trial for HAPE can help determine if HAPE is actually the problem. Have the victim stand quietly in a safe place and give him or her a 10 mg capsule of nifedipine, after puncturing it several times with a pin. Instruct the victim to chew and swallow the material. If the person subsequently feels faint, have him or her lie down. The victim may note easier breathing in ten minutes. If the person has not become profoundly faint and is breathing better, repeat the dose in fifteen minutes. If, after half an hour and two doses, the person's symptoms are noticeably better and if he or she has not fainted, give 20 mg of the slow-release (Adalat®) preparation every six hours. If you have the 30 mg long-acting preparation (Procardia XL®) give one or two tablets a day. Maintain hydration. You can stop the drug after a few days, or and when symptoms have been absent for twenty-four hours.

If the person becomes severely lightheaded or faint, put him on his back and elevate the legs to promote blood return to the heart. Do not give further nifedipine. When the individual is wide awake and can drink, give fluids. Don't allow him to stand unattended until he can do so without feeling lightheaded, and can walk unassisted. Do not give fluids by mouth to someone who is unconscious! Rely on other treatments for HAPE, especially descent, oxygen, or the hyperbaric bag.

By carrying and using a blood pressure cuff, you may reduce the likelihood of dosing someone with large amounts of nifedipine unnecessarily and causing adverse effects. You must be competent in its use, however. Measure the pressure before giving the drug and recheck it ten minutes after giving the first dose of 10 mg. If there is a drop of 10 mm or more in the diastolic pressure, and the person does not feel faint, repeat the dose in fifteen minutes as above. If there is no drop in blood pressure, similarly repeat the dose in fifteen minutes. If the person does feel faint, have him or her lie down, and repeat the first dose in thirty minutes instead of fifteen. If there is an improvement without severe lightheadedness, and the blood pressure drop hasn't been more than 20 mm, go ahead with the slow-release preparation as above. If there is a drop of more than 20 mm, give some fluids, and recheck the blood pressure in an hour. If the drop in the reading then is not more than 20 mm or the person feels faint or lightheaded, give the long-acting preparation.

Another monitoring method compares pulse readings standing and lying before and after giving the first dose of nifedipine. If, upon standing, there is a twenty point per minute rise and the person feels lightheaded, there is a significant postural drop in blood pressure. (This means the blood pressure standing is enough lower compared to sitting that the brain is being deprived of blood.) Get the person rehydrated and check the pulse changes again. If the drop is less than twenty, give the first dose of nifedipine and recheck the pulse changes lying and standing in fifteen minutes. Use pulse changes to guide further doses of nifedipine as if monitoring blood pressure.

The highly motivated climber or skier vacationing at a resort might contemplate further ascent if the treatment for HAPE was successful and certain conditions can be met. People have successfully reascended after recovery from HAPE—in circumstances where there was medical supervision in case problems recurred. If the illness was mild and the recovery swift, and if the victim was able to rest for a time at a lower altitude, you can consider reascending slowly with responsible companions; in this situation, nifedipine is also recommended. Read the protocols for health care providers (below) for guidelines.

The best experience with the nifedipine at present is in the European Alps. There, climbers have ascended rapidly, succumbed to HAPE, and recovered quickly when they have been speedily treated with nifedipine. Reports to date in the Himalaya, where ascent rates are usually slower, suggest that the response is protracted and not as dramatic. There is no central reporting scheme, so good experiences with it cannot be correlated with reports of it not working or causing serious side effects. Acetazolamide, in contrast, has been in use for over twenty-five years and has been evaluated by several controlled double-blind trials, the "gold standard" of assessment. We have a better understanding of what it can and probably cannot do.

Again, for children, there is no experience, but a dose of 0.25 mg/kg could be tried, twice a day, if in extenuating circumstances and if you can monitor the blood pressure.

## DEXAMETHASONE

This corticosteroid is recommended for treating anyone with severe symptoms of AMS and of HACE as an adjunct to the other therapies. Give 4 mg every six hours by mouth and begin with 8 mg as the first dose. If the victim is in a coma, the drug should be injected if possible. There is no need to place a tablet under the tongue. For children, if unable to descend, try a dose of 0.5 mg/kg every 6 hours.

## PAIN MEDICINE (ANALGESICS)

### NSAIDs ( Non Steroidal Anti Inflammatory Drugs)

These include aspirin (acetylsalicylic acid), acetaminophen (paracetamol), and ibuprofen, the commonest drugs of this class. There are myriad available by prescription in most countries. They can be used for headaches and the hangover-like symptoms in usual doses.

### Narcotics

Narcotics, including oxycodone, hydrocodone, meperidine, pethidine, morphine, and various others should not be used at altitude as they can depress respiration. Codeine in low doses (30 to 60 mg) may be safer.

## DIURETICS

When swelling of high altitude edema is severe enough to cause considerable discomfort and limit activity, a potent diuretic such as furosemide in small doses (20 or 40 mg orally) can be taken daily. The response is usually rapid. Give plenty of fluids. If there are signs of other than mild AMS, do not use this potentially hazardous therapy.

## ANTI-VOMITING MEDICINE

Prochlorperazine (Compazine® and other brands) would be the preferred drug to take, as it stimulates respiration, but it also can cause bizarre muscular side effects, so I would not recommend it. Promethazine is safer though it doesn't stimulate respiration. The rectal route is the preferred way to administer any anti-vomiting medicine. Consider injecting dexamethasone and descending if vomiting is severe.

## Adjunctive Treatment

Exhibiting compassion, establishing rapport with the victim, giving reassurance, listening actively, providing non-verbal support through touching, and showing concern are as important as other therapies. Reassure no matter how bleak the situation appears.

Rest is another treatment for mild HAPE. In high Andean clinical facilities, where oxygen was not available, rest has been successful. This is advisable only under medical supervision and where descent can be undertaken should the victim not respond.

One victim drained fluid from his lungs by essentially hanging upside down. (Consider it only under extreme conditions.) Some climbers advocate grunt breathing, or pursed lip breathing with cheeks puffed out, for mild HAPE. Complications of a collapsed lung or the induction of HACE are theoretically possible, so this method is not advised.

Some climbing doctors carry a CPAP (Continuous Positive Airway Pressure) mask, the kind with a deflatable ring seal, and tape a syringe to it for inflation, to temporize in treating HAPE.

# Treatment Protocols for Health Care Providers at Intermediate Altitudes

The following protocol is offered for medical people treating visitors to intermediate altitudes of 9,000 feet (2,750 m). This protocol should only be used in locations with rapid and reliable access to transportation, such as modern resorts or towns in developed countries. Medical people must administer the treatment and they must be quickly accessible to deal with problems that arise subsequent to treatment. The schema is given in clinical language, follows the principles of cost containment, and is the same as the protocol used at the clinic in Keystone, Colorado (9,200 ft. or 2,800 m).

AMS:
- If chest is clear on auscultation, then no chest film.
- Acetazolamide for sleep.
- Oxygen and rest for a severe headache, in addition to aspirin, ibuprofen, or acetaminophen.

HAPE:
- Vital signs by a nurse, including temperature (oral). There may be a hypertensive response, because of high norepinephrine release with HAPE.
- History and physical by a doctor.
- Pulse oximetry on room air (normal at Keystone is ninety to ninety-two percent and mild cases are between eighty and ninety percent, while readings in the seventies indicate severe HAPE).
- Oxygen by mask or nasal canula (flow rates of two to four liters per minute necessary to get oxygen saturation above ninety percent). If the saturation can't be raised to ninety percent with oxygen, then the victim needs to get to a hospital quickly.
- Chest film (may not be needed, but it can sometimes demonstrate unusual conditions, including cardiomegaly, pleural effusion).
- Pharmacotherapy of cases.
  - Nifedipine 10 mg, bitten and chewed, to see if there is a significant drop in blood pressure and if a clinical response is seen, then:

- Nifedipine 20 mg, long-acting, twice a day if no clinically significant hypotensive response.
- Four options (for those who wish to optimize a vacation).
  - If very sick (especially if confused), then evacuate by ambulance to a lower altitude.
  - If moderately sick (hypoxemia not readily corrected with oxygen), then hospitalize overnight, observe, keep on oxygen, monitor, and if better next day, send back to the hotel to rest and keep on oxygen.
  - If less sick (hypoxemia easily corrected with low flow oxygen), then send back to hotel (only if someone can be with the victim during the night) and get a hospital supply company to bring out oxygen; administer it by nasal prongs at two liters per minute all night. Check the next day and if patient is recovered to point of being asymptomatic, and if chest is clear to auscultation, rest a day and resume normal activity.
  - For very mild cases (just not feeling well, a few rales, small infiltrate on chest film, pulse oximetry above eight-five percent), send to hotel room, with nifedipine but without oxygen, and recheck the next day.
- If no response to nifedipine, then re-evaluate and evacuate patient.
- No use of furosemide.
- No CPAP, or PEEP, or grunt breathing.

HACE:
- Descent (ambulance evacuation).
- Oxygen.
- Dexamethasone (4 mg every six hours).
- Give diuretics such as furosemide if available.
- Consider mannitol and endotracheal intubation with hyperventilation.

# Chapter 6. Going to Altitude with a Preexisting Health Condition

As our population ages, more recognition is given to the beneficial physical, emotional, and psychological effects of exercise. More older people desire to travel to altitude for recreation. Some may be undertaking an altitude adventure for the first time in their lives; other seasoned travelers may have a chronic disease such as high blood pressure or diabetes. There are some published reports, but no controlled studies, of lowlanders with chronic diseases going to altitude. Not much is known about the effects of medicines at altitude, and advice by doctors to patients about their medication remains presumptive or speculative and patients should be cautious. In marginal clinical situations where a doctor has advised against taking an altitude sojourn, an individual who has a strong will and motivation to reach a personal goal might derive a far greater benefit from its attainment than from the loss of self-esteem resulting from staying at home in a low-risk environment and nursing the chronic illness.

If you have a chronic disease, such as high blood pressure, a heart condition, or diabetes, discuss the proposed altitude journey with your doctor. If your doctor is unfamiliar with the effects of altitude on your disease, refer her or him to the reading list for health workers in this book. Or, try to find an expert (see Where to Get More Information in Chapter 7). Your doctor working in conjunction with an altitude expert would be the best solution.

Some who should not venture to altitude, may wish to do so in spite of being advised against it by their doctors and experts. If you fall in the category of having a problem that will be made worse by altitude and want to go anyway, choose an itinerary with access to easy descent and medical help. Taking enough oxygen along is usually impractical but do bring a hyperbaric bag.

If you have a chronic disease that could cause problems at altitude, attempt a similar activity near home. Repeat the same effort at a moderate altitude (say 8,000 ft. or 2,450 m), also, hopefully, near home. If you perform well under both circumstances, consider that activity at even higher altitudes. The exercise guidelines for cardiac patients described under Heart Conditions, below, make sense for everyone.

The following advice is given regarding the more common chronic conditions affected by exposure to altitude.

## High Blood Pressure

Individuals with hypertension may find their pressures elevated at altitude because of increased activity of the sympathetic nervous system. Eat a low salt diet and schedule increased rest during the first few days at altitude. Seek advice from a knowledgeable physician regarding your medicines. If your blood pressure is difficult to control, either you or a companion should check it and be prepared to modify your drug regimen. Beta blockers, including propranolol, atenolol, and metoprolol, are probably not as effective at altitude as lower down. Clonidine and prazosin may be useful to control pressures. Other categories of drugs that may be useful at altitude include calcium channel blockers and ACE inhibitors, but there are no controlled studies of any drugs at altitude.

## Diabetes

Diabetics on insulin who have not traveled to a foreign country or undertaken the "planned adventure" should first take a shakedown trip to get used to monitoring blood sugars and modifying the insulin dose. Those on oral medicines are not subject to the same difficulties. Diabetics may experience problems regulating the insulin dose because of varying energy expenditure and food intake. More frequent blood glucose determinations and insulin dosing may be necessary. Shorter-acting preparations may make control easier. Carry glucagon and a few sugar cubes in case of insulin reactions. Companions need to be instructed in their use. Don't let insulin freeze and carry extra in case of loss or breakage. Control the blood sugar to have it in the slightly-higher-than-normal range, and do your best to not let your sugar get too high. Diabetics who have let their disease get out of control at altitude have had great difficulties in being treated for diabetic keto-acidosis, the extreme form of deranged sugar control.

## Neurologic Conditions

Transient ischemic attacks (TIAs) and strokes have been reported at high altitude (above 16,000 ft. or 4,900 m) in young healthy individuals. Dehydration may be a contributing factor. A TIA would be some brief neurologic difficulty, such as one side of the body or an arm or a leg being weak or numb. This would last more than a few minutes, but less than twenty-four hours. If you have such symptoms at altitude, then increase hydration, take an aspirin tablet a day and descend. If you have already had a stroke and recovered to function well enough to go to altitude, you can consider going. We know little about your risks in doing so.

If you have epilepsy and your seizures are controlled on medicines, be sure to continue your drugs at altitude. But if you have recently stopped your anti-seizure medicines at sea level because you hadn't had a seizure in a long time, your seizures may return after abrupt exposure to altitude.

The slight cerebral edema that develops at altitude may compromise the function of people with brain tumors. Tumors and other central nervous system conditions have first become symptomatic at altitude.

## Heart Conditions

If you have a heart condition, such as a previous heart attack or coronary bypass surgery, yet want to venture to altitude, don't despair. Many people do so successfully, and treasure the experience. Death while exercising does not appear more common at altitude than at sea level. What if you have no heart problems, but are worried about whether your heart can withstand going to altitude? If you are older, with risk factors for heart disease, then you might consult with your doctor who may suggest exercise testing, and if the results are positive, other studies. The exercise test, however, can be positive in normal people without heart disease and cause needless worry and expense. Argentinean authorities can require the results of an exercise test on anyone applying to climb Aconcagua.

Heart patients feel a sense of security in North America because they can dial 911 and be rapidly transported to modern emergency departments. In many altitude destinations throughout the world, help can be days away. Keep this in mind as you make your decision to go to such locations.

If you have angina and moderate symptoms, take a limited number of medicines, or have occasional angina at rest with some exercise limitations, then you may tolerate some exposure to altitude. If you have severe angina and limitation of physical effort at sea level, you are probably not reading this book. You should not go to altitude, as lack of oxygen there will increase cardiac work and precipitate severe attacks. If you are going to altitude with angina, ascend slowly, increase your anti-anginal medicines, and rest for the first 2–3 days on arrival there. Discuss treating significant blood pressure elevation using labetolol or clonidine with your doctor beforehand. Treat significant anginal symptoms with oxygen, if available, and descend without exertion.

If you have had a heart attack (myocardial infarction) and/or coronary bypass surgery, you need not be treated any differently than anyone in the above categories. You may have decreased exercise tolerance at altitude and have angina earlier. You are probably not at a greater risk of having another heart attack at altitude compared to performing the same exercise at sea level.

If you have somewhat controlled congestive heart failure (CHF) you may get worse at moderate altitude (6,500 ft. or 2,000 m) or higher. Determining whether your symptoms are due to your congestion getting worse or from mountain sickness may be difficult. AMS and fluid retention at altitude could aggravate your CHF, so avoid altitude.

Exercise guidelines at altitude are helpful for everyone. Maximal achievable heart rates decline at altitude whether or not you have heart disease. If you have coronary heart disease, having a target heart rate as an end point for activity levels at altitude is better than an activity prescription. From your treadmill test, your doctor can tell you what 75 percent of the ischemic end point heart rate at your home altitude would be. This is your target rate at altitude and would be reasonable for other individuals with chronic disease at altitude. Without an exercise study, you can substitute a derived maximal heart rate [maximal heart rate = 206 − 1.2(age − 20)] for the exercise study rate. Test this with strenuous exercise. Watches are available to measure your pulse.

See if you can maintain that heart rate comfortably. If not, scale it down to a rate you can.

## Lung Conditions

Many asthmatics report improvement in their condition at altitude, perhaps because there is less dust, a lower air density, and fewer inhaled allergens. There is a sanitarium at 10,500 feet (3,200 m) in Kyrgyzstan devoted to the clinical treatment of asthma! There, asthmatics benefit from taking acetazolamide (250 mg three times a day); the lower dose (125 mg) suggested here is probably as good before abrupt ascent and for one day afterward. Individuals with cold or exercise-induced asthma may have more attacks at altitude and should use inhaled bronchodilators before exposure.

Individuals with mild to moderate chronic lung disease (emphysema, or chronic bronchitis) may tolerate modest altitudes but are more likely to have AMS. Those on home oxygen should continue this and increase the flow rate by the ratio of the home to the new barometric pressure. If you have bad emphysema with marked lowering of oxygen in the arterial blood and retention of carbon dioxide, or sleep apnea, stay home. Those without a right pulmonary artery (don't ask me how anyone would *a priori* know this!) should be cautious about high altitude exposure, as their risk of HAPE is considerable.

## Blood Problems

If you have sickle cell disease, you shouldn't go to altitudes above 8,000 to 9,000 feet (2,440 to 2,740 m). Altitude exposures of only 6,320 feet (1,925 m) are associated with an almost 60 percent risk of crises. If you have sickle cell trait and other hemoglobinopathies such as SC or Hb S, ß+-thalassemia, but you have normal lung function, then limit exposure to 10,000 feet (3,050 m) and be aware that your spleen may give you problems. If you have a spleen (that has not previously become shrunken), then breathe supplemental oxygen during air travel (difficult on many airlines) and keep very well hydrated. If you have impaired lung function, problems may occur at altitudes lower than 10,000 feet (3,050 m).

The risk of blood clots is increased at altitudes above 14,000 feet (4,270 m), and possibly lower. Dehydration, increased blood counts, and inactivity while storm bound may increase the risk. The advisability of taking aspirin at altitude to prevent clots is discussed under Blood Response in Chapter 1.

## Obstetric and Gynecologic Conditions

While there is no evidence demonstrating that birth control pills cause blood clots at altitude, it could be a hazard. Women have been counseled to continue them at least to moderate altitudes (lower than 10,000 ft. or 3,000 m), as the risk of pregnancy may be greater than the possible increased risk of blood clots. Other experts disagree and advise the use of other contraceptives at altitude.

If you are pregnant and wanting to go to altitude, again, there is no data on which to base advice. The risk is probably greatest in the first three months. One lowlander is known to have climbed to an altitude of 24,600 feet (7,500 m) while four and a half months pregnant, and later gave birth to a "normal" child (who graduated from a top college). If you have concerns about the possible adverse effects of altitude on your unborn child, it is best not to go. Some experts advise against travel to altitude for the normal woman who is pregnant, while others would limit exposure to moderate altitudes (lower than 13,125 ft. or 4,000 m). A reasonable compromise would be to limit exposure during the first trimester to 8,000 feet (2,450 m) for uncomplicated pregnancies. If you have had great difficulties conceiving, don't go.

## Taking Your Children to Altitude

Infants and young children born at sea level are perhaps more at risk from altitude illness than adults. HAPE has been reported to be sixteen times more prevalent among children than adults in the Andes. If a child is not doing well at altitude it is more difficult to determine the cause. Children have been taken to altitudes over 15,000 feet (4,570 m) by responsible adults without incident. I would only advise this if the route permits rapid descent. Pharmaceuticals to prevent and treat altitude illness have not been studied in children, but dexamethasone and nifedipine doses are given for treatment in desperate situations. Acetazolamide can be used as well.

Children with bronchopulmonary dysplasia under 5 and those over 5 with pulmonary hypertension are at an increased risk of altitude illness, particularly HAPE. They should ascend very slowly. This also applies to those with cystic fibrosis. Children with cyanotic congenital heart disease (especially Tetralogy of Fallot) or those with a palliative procedure that depends on a low pulmonary vascular resistance should not go to altitude, nor should morbidly obese children.

## Miscellaneous Problems

### CONTACT LENSES

Extended-wear contact lenses have been worn to 26,250 feet (8,000 m) without mishap. Disposable lenses are advised as there are fewer risks of infection from improper cleaning. Gas permeable hard lenses have also been worn successfully. Bring plenty of "artificial tears" solution up high; the environment is very dry there. Eye-care materials and solutions are not available in many countries with high mountains. If there is any eye pain or redness while wearing contacts at altitude, remove them and instill antibiotic drops.

### ARTHRITIS

Joint problems should not behave any differently at altitude compared to sea level. Bilateral amputees have dragged themselves to lofty summits when their prostheses failed!

### CANCER

Cancer in remission or under control is not a reason to avoid altitude. Those who have had radiation to the neck may not do well at altitude.

### HIV/AIDS

The immune system that fights infection may not function well at altitudes above 10,000 feet (3,050 m). The HIV-infected traveler to altitude may have more serious problems with infections of the gastrointestinal tract. Choose a route or itinerary with an easy descent option because descent to a lower altitude would be the best choice if you suspect any infection.

## RADIAL KERATOTOMY

Individuals who have had corneal surgery to improve eyesight have experienced markedly decreased vision with exposure to increasing altitude. Overnight stays beginning at an intermediate altitude and going higher can result in a progressive shift toward farsightedness so that those who have had radial keratotomy may have difficulty recognizing people and distinguishing features of terrain. Secondary images may be observed. Changes are noticed at altitudes of 12,000 feet (3,600 m) and higher, usually after a 24-hour stay. Some people report changes at lower altitudes. Reading glasses may improve vision for those afflicted, but specific plus powers needed cannot be predicted in advance nor do they help the secondary images. Carry an assortment of reading glasses with different plus powers for temporary correction to allow safer descents if this occurs. Avoid hazardous routes and always be accompanied by someone without such corneal surgery. Problems with vision at altitude have not been reported to date in persons who have undergone photorefractive keratectomy, nor encountered in a study of such individuals.

## DIET PILLS

The weight-loss combination of fenfluamine and diethyproprion, called fen-fen, now off the market in the U.S., should not be taken by those going to altitude. I would caution against use of other diet pills as well.

# Chapter 7. Preparing to Go to Altitude

## Physical Preparation

To enjoy any activity at altitude, you need to get in good shape. Begin walking in hilly terrain with a small daypack. Increase the load and the duration of the exercise.

## Emotional Preparation

If you are mentally prepared for the activity and have a realistic self-appraisal and positive attitude, all will likely go well. The mental path depends on your own makeup and what you have done to prepare. Practicing meditation or following other relaxation programs, talking to people with experience in the activity, or seeking religion are effective means of preparation.

## Assembling a High Altitude Medical Kit

Even if you are going on a guided or organized trip to altitude, you should take responsibility for your own health. Some organized trips have sufficient supplies and knowledgeable personnel on them, but be prepared.

In addition to other medicines in the personal medical kit (see my book *The Pocket Doctor*), I advise anyone going to altitude to carry acetazolamide if they are not allergic to sulfas. If you are allergic and traveling independently, then carry dexamethasone. If you will camp above 12,000 feet (3,660 m)—this figure is somewhat arbitrary—then carry nifedipine and dexamethasone as well. If you have had HAPE before, carry nifedipine to any altitude. Consider renting a hyperbaric bag.

## Evaluating Modes of Travel to Altitude

If you are traveling to altitude with a commercial group, ask the company staff about the ascent profile, whether oxygen is carried, and whether a hyperbaric bag is taken. If you are paying for an expensive trip, one of the above should be included for sustained trips above 15,000 feet (4,575 m). Enquire about the content of the medical kit. What is the experience of the leader regarding success in taking clients to altitude? One guide regularly takes clients on treks to 21,000 feet and has remarkable success getting his charges there without incident. Ask to talk to clients who have been with your leader before to get a firsthand opinion of his or her capabilities. Talk to the guide directly. Ask about the altitude experience of other members of the group? Does the company screen its clients or just their wallets? What is the experience of the company in trips to high altitude? How often have they had to evacuate people? Have there been any fatalities? Ask to talk to clients who have been on trips where there have been evacuations to form an opinion of the company's safety interests?

What are the options for descent or evacuation at different places on the itinerary? Ask about contingency plans at various points on the ascent profile. For a journey to the Tibetan Plateau, where there are few options for descent, the answer is very important. Determine whether an individual who is not acclimatizing well can leave the group and be escorted down. Don't just take "Yes, of course" as an answer, but obtain details.

If you are going with friends on a non-commercial basis, discuss the contingency plans should someone get altitude illness. Decisions need to be made about whether the group wants to take a hyperbaric bag or oxygen along, and whether there will be communication options for rescue. The ease of descent is critical in choice of route.

If you are going with people you don't know well, get a sense of their priorities. Does a group member brag, "I'm going to make the summit or die trying"? When this individual gets in trouble with severe AMS, he or she may refuse to go down. Or, if you get sick, you could be abandoned.

If you are going solo, consider your route choices for descent and plan treatment options for altitude illness. What if there is no help nearby?

## Specific Situations

Common altitude environments and activities warrant discussion here. If you have had AMS before, plan to go skiing in one of the mountain states, live near sea level, will stay at a resort town above 6,000 feet, (1,830 m), and need to ascend quickly, consider taking acetazolamide. Commonly you fly to Denver and go on to Vail. Stay overnight in Denver, before going higher. Most people do well enough without taking acetazolamide. In one study, over half the people attending a conference in a hotel at an altitude of 9,800 feet (2,990 m) had symptoms of AMS. In another study at altitudes of 6,500 feet (1,980 m) a quarter of conference participants had symptoms of mild AMS. Although HAPE is relatively rare, hundreds of cases do occur each year in these places.

If flying to Lukla (9,200 ft. or 2,800 m) in Nepal, one starting point for the Everest Base Camp, do not try to get to Namche Bazaar (11,000 ft. or 3350 m) the first day. Follow the ascent guidelines and consider use of acetazolamide at night to improve sleep. If you have walked in from Jiri, you will do better. If landing in Lhasa (12,000 ft. or 3,660 m) or similar altitudes in South America, consider taking acetazolamide for prevention. If you haven't, use it when you arrive to treat symptoms of AMS and take it easy the first few days.

In climbing a mountain such as Rainier at 14,400 feet (4,390 m) in Washington State, people ascend to 10,000 feet (3,050 m) in one day, camp there and climb to the summit early the next morning. Most people suffer from AMS, although HAPE is almost unheard of unless people get stranded near the top and can't get down. Carry acetazolamide. It could be taken before bedtime to get better sleep. If you want to climb Kilimanjaro, try to arrive in Nairobi (5,500 ft. or 1,675 m) a few days early to acclimatize. Spend extra days at the higher huts on the ascent. This may be difficult because the guides there work against you as they herd people up. The ascent profile is rapid for most people, so consider taking acetazolamide at night, especially if you have had AMS before. If yours is a light alpine style expedition to 6,000 or 7,000+ meters (19,685 or 22965 ft.), carry acetazolamide, nifedipine, and dexamethasone, but use them only to treat altitude conditions. If you are climbing in the traditional expedition style by establishing a base camp at a high altitude, and your route lacks a quick, easy, rapid descent, take a hyperbaric bag and, possibly, oxygen.

Finally, if you are a member of a rescue party that is being helicoptered to 17,000 feet (5,200 m) on Mount McKinley to find a lost party, take both acetazolamide and dexamethasone before you depart and continue them during your stay up high.

## Where to Get More Information?

To learn more, attend conferences where experts talk on altitude illness and ask them questions. The Hypoxia Conference in the Canadian Rockies (http://www.hypoxia.net/), held in odd years in February, is one of the best. That web site as well as http://www.gorge.net/hamg/ and http://www.thebmc.co.uk/mm/mm0.html contain helpful resources. There are several conferences organized on wilderness medicine topics, including altitude illness, and presented for different types of audiences, often by outstanding faculty. Speak to doctors at travel medicine clinics to get referrals to other doctors knowledgeable about altitude illness. A travel clinic directory is at http://www.astmh.org/clinics/clinindex.html. Read sources in this book's bibliography. Talk to others who have been at altitude, ask local climbing clubs, and talk to people in outdoor/adventure equipment stores; the latter is the least reliable option.

# Chapter 8. Case Studies

The following are descriptions of situations where people had altitude illness, with accounts of how they were treated.

## SKIER AT U.S. ALTITUDE DESTINATION WITH HAPE

Reginald, a moderately obese thirty-year-old salesman from San Francisco, skied occasionally in the Lake Tahoe area. A late snowfall during a March cold spell tempted him to drive to Lake Tahoe (6,300 feet, 1920 m). The next day he skied at Heavenly Valley (between 7,000 and 10,000 ft. or 2,130 and 3,050 m). He drove to Mammoth (8,000 ft. or 2,440 m) where he spent the next two nights, and skied strenuously the next two days between 8,000 and 11,000 feet (2,440 and 3,350 m). He lost his appetite and did not drink much in the evenings at the bar, as he had done at Tahoe. On the afternoon of the second day at Mammoth, he was very short of breath and weak. He continued to ski, although by the end of the day he could barely get up the loading ramp to the lift. That night, he developed a cough, more shortness of breath, and a noisy chest. Medical help brought him to a hospital where HAPE was diagnosed, he was given nifedipine, and kept overnight on oxygen. Feeling normal the next day, he returned to his hotel and rested there, breathing oxygen obtained from a medical supply company. He was rechecked that evening and was told he could try skiing again if he continued taking nifedipine. He managed another day of skiing but was not the tiger he thought himself to be.

**Analysis.** Reginald had mild AMS that progressed to HAPE as he tried to be a weekend warrior. His obesity was a risk factor. With medical therapy, he recovered quickly and continued skiing. Victims at altitude resorts in developed countries where there is predictable rapid access to health care can salvage their vacations this way. Such a course would not be advisable, however, on a ski ascent of Broad Peak in the Karakorum (Pakistan). Reginald should be cautious about rapid ascents and vigorous activity at altitude in the future. A substantial loss of revenue results from people arriving at altitude resort destinations and not consuming expected quantities of food and beverages due to AMS. The industry is eager to see these vacationers treated for AMS!

## CLIMBER IN THE SIERRA WITH HAPE

Maureen, a twenty-four-year-old student, drove from sea level to a trailhead in the Sierra Nevada and slept at 8,000 feet (2,440 m). She was attempting to climb a 14,000-foot (4,270-m) peak over a long weekend. Maureen had slept at altitudes greater than 10,825 feet (3,300 m) on several similar climbing trips and had experienced mild AMS on half of those. She was in good physical shape, running twenty miles a week. She awoke with a headache and slight dizziness, but didn't tell her male companions and continued with them to 10,500 feet (3,200 m). Her headache improved with aspirin, but she slept fitfully. While climbing the following afternoon, she felt weak, became extremely short of breath ascending, and held the party back. Her headache got worse, and they bivouacked that night at 12,000 feet (3,650 m) without reaching the summit. She stated that her chest felt raspy, and she sensed gurgling there. In addition, she had a dry cough and couldn't sleep. The morning of her third day, Maureen's cough and headache was much worse, and she became very weak and had extreme difficulty breathing. She was helped down to 9,025 feet (2,750 m), while one of her partners headed out to get an air rescue. Maureen improved slightly that night. The next morning she was helicoptered out to a hospital at 4,200 feet (1,280 m). She was found to have X-ray changes typical of HAPE and recovered with oxygen.

**Analysis.** Easy, rapid access to high altitude is improving all over the world and is especially convenient in the Americas. Maureen's physical conditioning and goal orientation for this weekend climb allowed her to ascend rapidly. She denied the worsening symptoms of ascent. When she lost her ability to keep up with them, her companions should have got her down rather than bivouacking at altitude. Rapid ascents are best avoided in the future, and she should consider using nifedipine for prophylaxis.

## MCKINLEY CLIMBER WITH HACE

Kim, a thirty-four-year-old computer programmer from Korea came to climb Denali (20,320 ft. or 6,194 m) solo. He had previously climbed in the Alps. Kim ascended from the "Kahiltna International Airport"

(7,300 ft. or 2,225 m) and less than two days later, made camp at 14,000 feet (4,270 m) in a snow cave on the West Buttress route. The next day he was found by other climbers, stumbling and confused, but still attempting to ascend. They abandoned their ascent, gave him dexamethasone, acetazolamide, and nifedipine, and took turns carrying and dragging him down. His breathing did not improve much as they struggled to get him to 10,000 feet (3,050 m). However, they were able to complete the evacuation to the "airport" and by then his symptoms had cleared. He couldn't remember what had happened and wanted to continue his ascent, but his rescuers' opinions prevailed and he was flown out.

**Analysis.** The ascent rate in this highly motivated climber was far too rapid. He developed HACE and was lucky that climbers were nearby, and willing to help. The treatment was shotgun, as is often the case in desperate situations. Getting an ataxic climber down on a big mountain is challenging.

## TREKKER TO MOUNT EVEREST WITH FATAL HAPE

Robert, a forty-one-year-old engineer, was a member of "The Highest Trek in the World" to Camp 3 (20,800 ft. or 6,340 m) on Everest. He had previously climbed Kilimanjaro (19,340 ft. or 5,895 m) and wanted to get above 6,000 meters (19,685 ft.). Because of a delayed business deal, he flew to Lhasa (12,000 ft., 3,660 m) two days behind his trekking party. After two nights in Lhasa, Robert hired a jeep to catch up with the group. He avoided medicines on religious grounds and did not take any acetazolamide. He was driven to the Everest Base Camp (16,900 ft. or 5,150 m) in 3 days. Upon arrival at the Base Camp, he was found to have a severe headache and nausea. The jeep departed. Against his wishes, he was given 500 mg of acetazolamide, but the next morning the symptoms continued and he vomited several times. The trip leader felt the vomiting was due to the large dose of acetazolamide and gave him another medicine for vomiting. He suggested Robert descend on a yak, but Robert refused, saying he would be fine after a night's sleep. That night he had a non-productive cough for which he was given some cough medicine. He awoke with extreme shortness of breath, and was diagnosed with HAPE. Another party there, about to descend, had a Gamow Bag® and he was put into it for a total of three hours. After the first two hours, he asked to come out of the bag and became breathless again. He spent another hour inside it and came out of the bag much better. The other party descended with the bag. Robert felt too sick to continue up to Camp 3, but said he would improve at base camp. His party proceeded with their scheduled itinerary, leaving later that day while an attendant remained with him. That night, he slept in the tent by himself, and in the morning he was found dead.

**Analysis.** It is nearly impossible to avoid rapid transport to significant heights in Tibet. Hurried vacations, demanding itineraries, and the difficulties in arranging a quick rescue are some of the hazards of travel there. This case illustrates some of the realities of commercial trips. In an attempt to achieve his goal, Robert ascended far too quickly. Once severe AMS was diagnosed, descent options were limited and, in an attempt to please the client, the leader did not require him to go down. The victim of altitude illness is rarely competent to make decisions about his care. Continued access to the Gamow Bag® was problematic. Descent should have been undertaken by yak or porter, and he should not have been allowed to sleep in the tent alone.

## TREKKER TO MOUNT EVEREST WITH FATAL HAPE

George, a sixty-two-year-old doctor had been evacuated from Mount Kenya in February with HAPE that improved immediately on descent. He was found to have high blood pressure and was put on medicine for that. In the spring, he walked from Jiri (6,250 ft. or 1,905 m) to Gorakshep (17,000 ft. or 5,185 m) in Nepal's Everest region in ten days. He developed a dry cough and his medical companion gave him a furosemide injection during an attempted descent. An air rescue was launched and three days later he ended up in a Kathmandu hospital, where he continued to be short of breath and blue in spite of oxygen treatment. He deteriorated and died twenty-six hours after admission there, despite heroic attempts to treat him. At autopsy, he had findings of severe HAPE.

**Analysis.** There was no attempt to prevent HAPE by taking nifedipine, the ascent rate was too fast, descent was delayed waiting for an air evacuation, and the medical treatment in the field was inappropriate. In spite of descent to a lower altitude, he deteriorated, probably because the initial HAPE process, which was a lung injury, had progressed to irreversible lung disease as confirmed by autopsy. In the one study of autopsy findings on seven trekkers dying of altitude illness in Nepal, three were physicians!

## HIMALAYAN CLIMBER WITH AMS AND HAPE

Albert, a thirty-two-year-old teacher, flew from Kathmandu to Lukla (9,200 ft. or 2,800 m) and took 500 mg of acetazolamide daily to prevent AMS. He continued on to a base camp of 17,700 feet (5,400 m) in three days, arriving with a significant headache and loss of appetite. He joined two friends there, who had just climbed a trekking peak in the Khumbu, and the three planned to undertake a demanding alpine ascent. In two days they reached 22,640 feet (6,900 m) where they camped. During the night, Albert developed shortness of breath and a rapidly worsening cough. In the morning he was extremely short of breath, coughing, and almost unable to get out of the tent. His companions recognized that he had HAPE, and gave him 10 mg of nifedipine. In fifteen minutes, Albert felt his breathlessness was slightly better, and he coughed less. He was soon able to slowly ascend 300 feet (100 m) and traverse over to an easier descent route. There he took 20 mg of the slow-release preparation of nifedipine and descended to the base camp on his own. That night, at the 6,900 meter camp, he again had another episode of HAPE, which he treated with 20 mg of nifedipine under the tongue, followed by 20 mg of the slow-release preparation. He was able to descend to 5,000 meters (16,400 ft.) the next day and had no further respiratory problems. He did not resume his climb.

**Analysis.** This case demonstrates that taking acetazolamide neither prevents HAPE nor masks the symptoms of it. Flights to altitude are always more risky instead of gradual ascents. The dose of acetazolamide was higher than necessary. Acetazolamide does not guarantee that you won't get AMS, it just lessens the chances. After ascending too quickly, he joined friends who were already acclimatized. Climbing alpine style presents further risks, especially to inexperienced climbers who don't take enough time for acclimatization. Albert did not rest or do short day climbs when he had symptoms of AMS. His continued ascent profile was too rapid. HAPE was treated in the field with nifedipine which allowed him to descend without the problems of trying to carry out a rescue. Besides a more gradual ascent in the future, Albert should take nifedipine to prevent recurrence of HAPE.

## KILIMANJARO CLIMBER WITH SEVERE AMS

Gail, a forty-year-old nurse in good physical condition, had climbed to the summit of Mount Whitney (14,494 ft. or 4,418 m) two months before she went to Kilimanjaro. Her group followed a standard strategy for the climb of "Kili," Africa's highest peak at 19,340 feet (5,895 m). After spending the night in Marangu, 4920 feet (1500 m), a subtropical oasis, they hiked to Mandara Hut (8,860 ft. or 2,700 m), rested, and spent the night. They went on to Horombo Hut (12,200 ft. or 3,720 m) where they spent two nights before continuing up to Kibo Hut at 15,420 feet (4,700 m). Gail kept up a good pace throughout. She felt fine and did not take acetazolamide, although other members of her group did. Reaching Kibo, she felt some shortness of breath and slowed her pace, but did not become seriously ill. Next morning, on the attempt to reach the summit, Gail started out strong, but fell behind after two hours. She was ataxic, had difficulty breathing, and had to stop to rest after every step, in spite of supreme effort to keep going. Her condition deteriorated rapidly. She began to vomit and was forced to turn back several hundred feet short of Gilman's Point on the edge of the crater. Gail descended to Kibo Hut with her guide's assistance and then on to Horombo. Within a couple of hours, she felt fine again.

**Analysis.** Gail had attempted to pre-acclimatize on Whitney, but there is little residual effect after two months. A week's stay in Leadville, Colorado (10,170 ft. or 3,100 m) just prior to departure would have been better. She most likely had mild HACE which usually clears rapidly with descent. HAPE can take much longer to resolve, especially if it has been present for some time. In many situations both HACE and HAPE are both present, though one can be sub-clinical, that is, there is a disorder present, but symptoms are not noticeable.

## CLIMBING ACONCAGUA AFTER CARDIAC BYPASS SURGERY

Harry, an experienced fifty-one-year-old climber/lawyer, underwent coronary artery bypass surgery a year after a heart attack. He had recovered fully and was symptom free, exercising regularly and climbing peaks near home. He wanted to fulfill his dream of climbing Aconcagua, the highest summit in the Americas (22,834 ft. or 6,960 m). His doctor advised him against it, and he subsequently had a clinical depression. He sought out advice at a meeting of altitude researchers. A lively debate ensued, and he realized there was no strong consensus among the experts. He accepted the risk of being far from help should problems arise, joined a commercial climb that included a climbing doctor, and informed the others on the expedition of his condition. A treadmill test was done as required by the Argentinian authorities. He prepared by exercising in Colorado around 10,000 feet (3,050 m) for a week before departure and perfected pacing himself with his target heart rate. During the trip to base camp he took acetazolamide, and monitored his blood pressure. He avoided strenuous carries for the first few days, then began humping moderate loads and watched his pace by monitoring his pulse. He experienced no unexpected problems. Bad weather prevented them from reaching the summit, but he did reach the team's high point of 20,000 feet (6,095 m) without incident. Upon arrival back home, his mood remained good. Although he has no desire to return to Aconcagua, he continues moderate climbs.

**Analysis.** A reasoned person may accept risks and behave in a responsible manner towards his climbing companions. Some trekkers and climbers have not told their partners on a venture about their chronic illness, then deteriorated up high and imposed an unexpected burden on the others.

# Chapter 9. Questions and Answers

Some people find they learn better by asking questions than by reading text.

## General Issues About Altitude

*I've never been to altitude before. What should I worry about in going there?*

Nothing! Going to altitude is a pleasurable experience providing you don't ascend too quickly. Do pay attention to changes in your functioning and monitor how tired you are, including recovery time from an activity. If you are not doing so well, don't raise your sleeping altitude until you are better. If this doesn't work, go down to below the altitude at which you first noticed any symptoms of altitude illness.

*Is good physical fitness protective for altitude illness?*

No. Fit individuals may experience more altitude illness because such they can go higher more quickly. Fit people find it easier to enjoy activities at altitude. They should not try to compete with high altitude natives, such as Sherpas, who are in their element.

*What is a good pace at altitude?*

One that does not exhaust you and allows you to walk all day without extreme fatigue. A common beginner's mistake is to walk too quickly and make frequent rest stops. Follow a rate of activity that does not require you to rest every fifteen minutes or half an hour. Learn the rest step for climbing: position your foot for your next step and before bearing weight on it, rest it briefly. Then shift your weight and repeat the process. Synchronize your breathing with your climbing. Low down, on steep ascents, inhale on one step and exhale on the next. Higher, inhale and exhale on every step. At extreme altitudes, take two or three breaths with every step, at a rhythm that you can continue without stopping to rest. Repeat a verse of a song or a mantra in synchrony with your feet and lungs. Vary the pace depending on the trail and conditions of the climb. Speed up on easier sections, slow down on more strenuous. Begin the day's journey slowly, and as the muscles and cardiovascular system have "stretched," increase the pace. Toward the end of the day, slow down.

The other less common mistake people make is to walk too slowly, which is fatiguing in itself. Walk at your own pace and not that of the person in front of you. A certain level of discomfort in exercising at altitude (and at sea level) must be tolerated.

### What is the safe daily rate of ascent at altitude?

No rate is safe for all. Published itineraries for groups going to high altitude on commercial or private trips, will be too fast for perhaps ten or twenty percent of the participants. Not raising the sleeping altitude more than 1,000 feet (300 m) a day above 10,000 feet (3,050 m) is offered as a safe rate of ascent, if a stopover day is thrown in for every 2,000 or 3,000 feet (609 or 1,000 m) of altitude gained. On the stopover day, climb as high as you like but return to the previous night's altitude to sleep. Some people will find this too fast, so if they get AMS, those individuals should slow down.

### What is the finger test for altitude?

The finger test is a procedure to measure the oxygen saturation of the arterial blood, using a modern device called a pulse oximeter, in which a sensor is attached to the end of a finger. The reading represents the percentage of hemoglobin in the arterial blood that is saturated with oxygen. As one climbs higher, less oxygen is available to fill the oxygen-binding sites on the hemoglobin molecule. Newcomers to altitude have lower readings that increase with acclimatization. Individuals with HAPE will have significantly lower readings. At sea level, the normal reading is 96 percent or above, while at 15,000 ft (4572 m) it is around 86 percent, dropping to about 76 percent around 20,000 ft (6096 m). At the summit of Everest, 29,029 ft (8848 m), it drops to approximately 58 percent.

Some groups at altitude carry a pulse oximeter with them, attempting to gauge how well individuals are acclimatizing and hoping to diagnose HAPE with the instrument. Foreign climbers have recently arrived at the 14,000-ft level (4627-m) level on Denali, where there is sometimes a park ranger stationed, and asked for the "finger test." Cold fingers can give falsely low readings, as can strenuous exercise. I feel there is no reason to carry such an expensive device and encourage people to use the principles discussed in this book instead.

*If I have altitude illness, does that mean that I will never be a successful high altitude climber?*

No. It is okay to have altitude illness. Many Everest summiters have had HAPE and HACE. It is not okay to die from altitude illness, a preventable condition that results in total recovery, if diagnosed and treated early enough.

*I had HAPE before at 14,000 feet (4,270 m). Does that mean I will always get it at this altitude?*

No, it varies with each excursion to altitude. If you ascend slowly enough, you will not get it.

*I've tried to climb Mount Rainier numerous times and find that I always get stopped at 12,000 feet (3,660 m) and can't seem to get higher. Is there a ceiling for certain individuals at altitude?*

Perhaps. Try acetazolamide before and during the ascent, and spend an extra day or two at the lower camp before attempting the summit.

*Are men more likely to get altitude illness than women?*

More victims are male, but more men go to altitude. Women tend to breathe more at altitude than men suggesting they may be less susceptible to HAPE. Menstruation in women is probably not a risk factor for getting altitude illness. Also women are less macho, silent, and goal oriented, which works in their favor. These being the 1990s, everyone's at risk.

*Should I take birth control pills at altitude?*

Yes, if you need them for contraception. There is no evidence that it is harmful to take them, although on theoretical grounds oral contraceptives may increase the risk of blood clots higher up.

*Is consuming alcohol bad for acclimatization at altitude?*

Probably. The early symptoms of altitude illness resemble those of a hangover. By imbibing, it may be difficult to tell whether you are suffering from altitude illness or from the effects of alcohol. Alcohol depresses respiration during sleep. Avoid alcohol until you are well acclimatized and not going higher.

*Can judgment be impaired at altitude?*

Yes. Psychometric studies on individuals at high altitude show a loss of performance.

*I'm going to altitude with a commercial group that is carrying a hyperbaric bag. Doesn't that lessen my chances of having problems with serious altitude illness?*

No. It is unclear whether a group carrying a hyperbaric bag is less likely to have problems. Among trekkers to high altitude destinations in Nepal, those traveling independently are less likely to experience a fatality resulting from altitude illness (see Shlim, 1992). Such people may be more flexible in their schedules and less likely to have peer pressure operating. The bag may not change that. Aggregate statistics do not distinguish between groups with experienced, competent leaders, and those without. Travelers with commercial groups should assess the competence of their leaders as there are no regulatory standards.

*I feel myself suffocating and not sleeping well at altitude. I catch myself falling asleep and suddenly waking up, feeling claustrophobic in the tent. What should I do?*

Avoid sleeping pills and take acetazolamide at bedtime.

*I live at sea level. Are my chances of getting AMS greater than someone who lives at 5,000 feet (1,525 m) or higher?*

    Yes.

*Up high, I lose all my sexual drive. Is this normal?*

    Yes, although others report an increase libido, an erotic hypoxia.

# Pharmacologic Prevention and Therapy

*I'm going to altitude. Should I take acetazolamide to prevent altitude illness?*

    No, unless one of the following applies: you have predictably and repeatedly had altitude illness before; you are on a specific time-cramped itinerary; or you are flying to destinations such as Lhasa, Tibet.

*At what altitude should I start to take acetazolamide for preventing altitude illness, given that I have decided to take it?*

    Just before any abrupt increase in altitude above 8,000 feet (2,450 m). Begin the day you ascend.

*How much acetazolamide should I take for prevention of altitude illness?*

    Take 125 mg (half a tablet) twice a day, morning and night.

*Can taking acetazolamide mask the symptoms of altitude illness?*

    No.

*I'm allergic to sulfa drugs. Should I take any other drug for preventing altitude illness?*

    Allergic reactions to acetazolamide are rare. People ascribe many different symptoms to allergies. If you have a supposed allergy to sulfa drugs, consult your doctor. Consider taking a test dose of acetazolamide under a controlled clinical situation to determine whether or not you have a true allergy. Dexamethasone is not recommended for preventing altitude illness in routine situations. Consider it for rescue situations to high or extreme altitude requiring rapid ascent by air transport. Take nifedipine if you have had HAPE before.

*Will I get rebound altitude illness if I stop taking acetazolamide?*
     No. It actually aids acclimatization. Stopping dexamethasone, the other prophylactic, can result in rebound illness.

*I'm taking acetazolamide, so I can't get HAPE or HACE, right?*
     Wrong. Many people have succumbed to HAPE, HACE, and AMS while taking acetazolamide. Only the chances of getting AMS are decreased.

*I read the package insert on acetazolamide. So many side effects are listed. Which ones are commonly reported at altitude?*
     Every side effect ever reported is listed in the manufacturer's statement. Tingling of the lips, fingers, and toes is common, as is having to urinate more. It also changes the taste of carbonated beverages, although many people don't report this.

*Acetazolamide, by your accounts, is a great drug. Why not recommend everyone take it at altitude?*
     I believe in avoiding drugs if there are equally effective alternatives, such as slow ascent. If you believe in a pill for every ill, you may want to act differently. Many people find the tingling it causes annoying.

*My friends are trying to get me to take dexamethasone whenever we climb above 14,000 ft (4627 m), saying it makes them feel great and perform better. What do you think?*
     Some people feel dexamethasone, a steroid, is a wonder drug. The controlled double-blind studies, in which recipients didn't know whether they were getting it or a placebo, did not show this to be so. Dexamethasone does prevent AMS, but does not aid acclimatiza-

tion, as acetazolamide does—acetazolamide both prevents and treats AMS. Steroids can cause euphoria or depression. If your pills were to get lost or avalanched off, you would be in deep trouble. The side-effect profile does not warrant even thinking of using this drug routinely. Competitive athletes are disqualified if found to be using this pharmacologic agent; should climbers be any different?

*My doctor suggested my taking a sleeping pill since restful sleep is said to be hard to come by at altitude. There is nothing wrong with that, is there?*

Yes, there is. Sleeping pills were routinely prescribed by doctors a few decades ago to insure a good sleep at altitude. Because they depress respiration, a critical factor in acclimatization, taking sleeping pills, sedatives, or tranquilizers is dangerous.

*Now that there is a drug to treat HAPE, isn't altitude illness a less serious problem?*

Nifedipine has received attention because of its reported ability to help symptoms of HAPE. Studies done by Oswald Oelz and Peter Bärtsch, among others, have shown nifedipine to be very useful in preventing HAPE on rapid ascents of Monta Rosa in the Alps. The treatment effect has not been subjected to a controlled trial. It does not appear to be as dramatic in HAPE that comes on during slower ascents in the Himalaya. People have died, presumably from HAPE, after taking nifedipine.

*Aspirin has been touted as panacea for extending life and preventing heart attacks. Should I take it at altitude?*

Maybe. If you take it on a regular basis at home, then continue this at altitude. Whether or not aspirin really is beneficial in sojourners to altitude is unknown. There are theoretical grounds for taking it, at least at extreme altitude (above 18,000 ft. or 5,500 m), but it doesn't make sense for everyone at altitudes below that. Discuss this with an altitude-aware doctor.

*What about taking furosemide and other potent diuretics at altitude?*

Don't. Initial studies supported their use in preventing altitude illness. They have not been repeated successfully and there is no justification for using them at present. Significant side effects, including dehydration and fainting, result from their use. Faced with a serious case of HAPE, most clinicians who carry the drug will likely administer it.

*Do antacids prevent altitude illness?*

No. Experiments testing the hypothesis did not show any effect.

# Diet and Hydration Related to Altitude Illness

*Is there a special diet that is to be recommended at altitude?*

While on theoretical grounds, a low-fat, low-salt, and high carbohydrate diet could be best, there are few dietary options for those visiting high altitudes and eating locally produced foods. Eating very salty foods has been reported to increase the risk of altitude illness. A good appetite is a sign of adaptive acclimatization at altitude, so eat what appeals to you and is convenient to prepare. The widely touted high-energy foods may not be palatable up high. Besides being very expensive, they freeze solid in the cold of high altitude. Thin people may welcome some fat in the diet to help keep insulation from melting away.

*Will keeping well hydrated prevent altitude illness?*

Hydration by itself will probably not prevent altitude illness. One can easily get dehydrated at high altitude because the ambient air is so dry and activity increases insensitive loss. Dehydration may increase the risk of developing altitude illness. Drinking enough water requires effort at altitude, to melt snow or to purify a liquid source, but trip leaders report that keeping well hydrated is an important factor for success. In some parts of the world, people are advised not to drink water during the day's activities, but to hydrate before and after. The timing of hydration has not been adequately studied, but I advise frequent hydration.

Soup mixes, drink powders, instant eggnog, cider, cocoa, herbal teas, and so forth make water more palatable and easier to consume in quantity at altitude.

*All this talk about hydration, when the syndromes to be feared most are excess water in the brain and the lungs. Shouldn't we be drinking less?*

No. Waterlogging of brain or lungs is not a problem of water overload, but of leakage from spaces where water is to where it shouldn't be. The lack of oxygen in cells causes this, not an excess of water.

*I'm incredibly thirsty at high camp, but have lost my water purification materials. Can I drink the water here anyway?*

Yes. Treating significant dehydration when it occurs, takes precedence over the cleanliness of the water source. Melted snow is safe enough as are mountain water sources without a population center or animals nearby. There are heavily trafficked areas such as the "Kahiltna International Airport" or the foot of the Khumbu Icefall where I advise caution. Do not wait for thirst to signal the need to drink; this mechanism may not work well up high.

## Effects of Altitude Illness

*I went on a trek to altitude in Nepal and wasn't feeling well. I don't recall the details, but a helicopter was called and I was evacuated. When I arrived in Kathmandu, I felt perfectly fine. I should not be liable to pay the rescue bill, since I really wasn't sick there. Isn't it up to the agency and the trek leader to pay for it?*

You should gratefully pay for being alive. Such common stories indicate the person had a form of altitude illness requiring descent that was promptly carried out resulting in a rapid response and a survivor. The leader should be thanked for exercising conservative judgment which is prudent at altitude. There are too many situations where people waited too long, and bodies were evacuated. Inquire from your travel agent about rescue insurance before you leave.

*I feel awful and it's getting dark. Can't I wait until morning to get down?*

No. You are faced with a difficult decision. There are too many cases where a corpse was found in the morning to even suggest waiting.

*I walked slowly from Lukla to Namche Bazaar and I still got altitude illness. What should I do differently on my next trip to altitude?*

It is not the speed of your walking, but the amount that you raise your sleeping altitude that counts. Sleep at Lukla the first night and at Jorsale the next, before ascending to Namche. Do not carry a loaded pack the next time to limit exertion as those who exercise at a more rapid rate may be more inclined to get AMS and HAPE.

*Couldn't my breathing condition, cough, and fever, be pneumonia at altitude? Shouldn't I wait to see if the antibiotics work?*

No. Best to treat all suspected cases of pneumonia at altitude as if they were HAPE and add an antibiotic to the regimen.

*My Sherpa, Lhakpa, has rapid breathing, lethargy, and cough. A high altitude native, he couldn't have HAPE, could he?*

Yes, he could have HAPE and he needs to be treated as any other person with the same symptoms. Some lowlanders in Nepal call themselves Sherpa to get the business.

*Could my diarrhea be a symptom of altitude illness?*

Unlikely. Your water losses increase at altitude, so hydrate more.

*I've had a cold, which started before coming to altitude. Now the trip leader is concerned that I have HAPE. My symptoms seem the same. Could she be right?*

Yes. Others are often more capable than you to notice changes in signs of altitude.

*The trek leader listened to my lungs and told me she heard rales. Does this mean I have HAPE?*

No, rales are common at altitude, and do not by themselves mean a person has HAPE. If rales (also called crackles) persist after several deep breaths, HAPE or a pneumonia could be present. Look for other signs and symptoms.

*My companions say I have HAPE. I have descended a thousand feet to where I first began to feel the extreme shortness of breath. Now I feel a little better. Should I spend the night here and see how I feel in the morning?*

No. Such a scenario has proven fatal. When you have serious symptoms of altitude illness, you should descend to below the altitude at which you first had any symptoms of altitude illness, even mild ones. You may not improve significantly before doing so.

*Everyone in my group, except me, got up several times last night to pee. I feel fine, what should I do? Drink more?*

Yes, you may well be dehydrated. Check for other symptoms of altitude illness as well, and act accordingly. Alert your companions that you are not urinating as much as them. Ask that they watch you for possible signs of developing altitude illness.

*We were all short of breath ascending to the high point. Why all this fuss about me, continuing to be short of breath?*

The key point is whether or not you improved with rest. Those short of breath with activity should get better quickly with rest.

*I've climbed ten 14,000-foot or higher peaks in Colorado. That means I'll have no problems from altitude going to Everest Base Camp, right?*

Unfortunately, no. Response to altitude is variable from person to person and from trip to trip. There are many Everest summiters who have since had serious symptoms of altitude illness at much lower elevations.

*I'm a doctor, I know what is going on, and I do not have altitude illness!*

The mortality rate for doctors at high altitude is disproportionately high.

*I notice that George in the next tent is short of breath all the time, even when resting. He eats very little at meals. He says he's fine. Should the rest of our group be concerned or take action?*

Yes. It could be altitude illness denial. Go through the protocol and act accordingly, or get George down a few thousand feet and see if he improves.

*Sandra has been getting worse at altitude for the last few days. The leader says it is because she has the flu, is dehydrated, and hasn't been practicing her meditation exercises properly. What should we do?*

Act on humanitarian grounds and get the leader to agree to have her descend without delay to see if she improves. If the leader refuses, consider going against the decision.

*Jeremy has died in Dolpo of presumed altitude causes. Shouldn't we do all we can to get the body back to his home?*

No. Recognize how difficult it is to transport a corpse on carriers in many countries, impossible in some. A proper traditional disposal of the remains according to the local custom should be considered. You will need to deal with local authorities and other survivors. Write down what happened, photograph everything, and save as many personal effects as possible.

## Who Should Go to Altitude?

*I'm pregnant, and want to go on a high altitude adventure. Is this wise?*

We do not know about the effects of altitude on pregnancy to either the lowlander mother or the fetus. If there was a mishap in the pregnancy outcome that could be attributed to altitude, would you blame yourself? Then limit altitude exposure to 10,000 to 12,000 feet (3,050 to 3,660 m), so you don't seriously compromise the amount of oxygen carried in the blood. A miscarriage in a remote area would be scary for most women.

*Should I take my children to high altitude with me?*

As more and more parents venture to altitude, children accompany them to altitudes of 18,000 feet (5,500 m) or so, without ill effect. A leisurely itinerary is important. Children aged 3 and 7 have hiked to the top of Kala Pattar (18,500 ft.or 5,640 m). A 3 1/2 year old was successfully treated for symptoms of lethargy in a Hyperbaric Bag. It is difficult to identify symptoms and signs in children as altitude illness. Altitude localities are cold and remote, making evacuation worrisome. Consider any questionable behavior at altitude to be altitude illness. If you descend quickly, few problems should result.

*Does it make sense to postpone the trip to altitude for a few years until we know more about the scourge of altitude illness?*

At present, we know what we need to in order to prevent deaths from altitude illness.

*I have heart disease and other medical problems, including having had coronary bypass surgery. I take medicines for high blood pressure. My doctor says I shouldn't even think of going to Khumbu to see Mount Everest, though it has been a lifelong dream of mine. Should I listen to him?*

The answer depends on the benefits that you will gain from attaining your goal weighed against the increased risk in being in a place where full service emergency care is not minutes away. The chance of dying from heart disease does not appear higher at altitude than at sea level. If you decide to go, find a doctor who can advise you to modify your blood pressure drugs at altitude if necessary. Travel with a group that includes altitude savants.

*Are individuals with migraine headaches more inclined to migraine headaches at altitude?*

Yes. Treat them as any other headache at altitude, checking for ataxia, rapid breathing, and so forth. Don't ascend, and try pain medicine if there are no ominous findings.

# Glossary

*Acclimatization:* The process of the body adapting to high altitude where there is less oxygen in the air to breathe.

*Acute Mountain Sickness (AMS):* In the setting of a recent gain in altitude, the victim experiences a headache and at least one of the following symptoms:

- Gastrointestinal problems (poor or no appetite, nausea or vomiting)
- Fatigue or weakness
- Dizziness or lightheadedness
- Difficulty sleeping

*Altered mental status:* A change in the level and functioning of the psyche (a person's intellectual functioning, including his or her emotional state, attitude, psychological condition, and personality aspects). The affected individual is not thinking clearly and he or she may not be aware of external events or surroundings.

*Altitude illness:* The totality of problems associated with not feeling well at altitude.

*Ataxia:* Altered balance and muscular coordination resulting from the brain not working correctly. Check for ataxia by performing the tandem walking test (see Chapter 4, section III).

*Cyanosis:* A bluer skin color than that of similarly complexioned companions, reflecting the inability to transport oxygen adequately in the blood (in daylight, compare the color of lips or fingernail beds).

*Disease:* Literally a lack of ease, but understood as a disorder of physiological or psychological function in the biomedical model.

*Diuresis:* An increase in urination.

*Extreme altitude:* Elevations above 18,000 feet (5,500 m).

*High Altitude Cerebral Edema (HACE):* In the setting of a recent gain in altitude, the presence of a change in mental status and/or ataxia in a person with AMS or the presence of both mental status change and ataxia in a person without AMS.

*High Altitude Edema:* Swelling of the hands, face, or ankles at altitude.

*High Altitude Pulmonary Edema (HAPE):* In the setting of a recent gain in altitude, the presence of at least two of the following signs and symptoms.

Symptoms:

- Shortness of breath at rest
- Cough
- Weakness or decreased exercise performance
- Chest tightness or congestion

Signs:

- Rales or wheezing in at least one lung field
- Central cyanosis
- Rapid breathing
- Rapid heart beat

*High Altitude Retinopathy:* Changes in the retina of the eyes at altitude, in which there is bleeding and other pathology.

*High Altitude Syncope:* Fainting that occurs after eating and standing up a day after arrival to moderate altitudes. The faint is followed by quick recovery.

*Illness:* A state of feeling unwell.

*Intermediate altitude:* Defined in this book as altitudes to 12,000 feet (3,660 m).

*Periodic breathing:* During sleep, cyclical changes in the rate and depth of breathing from rapid and strong to weak and almost imperceptible.

*Sickness:* A role bestowed upon an individual by a community or group characterized by some deficit in normal mental or physical function.

*Sign:* What is externally observable in a sick person, usually taken to mean what a health practitioner sees, feels, listens to, or measures.

*Symptoms:* What a sick person feels or complains about.

*Syncope:* Denoting a brief loss of consciousness termed a faint.

*Syndrome:* An association of symptoms and signs that occur together more often than would be expected by chance.

*Tandem walking test:* A test for ataxia (see Chapter 4, section III).

# Table 1 Symptoms and Signs

| Symptom | Description | Indicator of | What to do |
|---|---|---|---|
| headache | | AMS<br>HACE | • painkillers, rest; re-evaluate in 12 hours<br>• look for other symptoms<br>• do not raise sleeping altitude |
| shortness of breath | | AMS<br>HAPE | • see if this stops with rest; if not treat for HAPE |
| cough | | HAPE<br>and many other problems | • very common at altitude and due to many causes besides altitude, including dry air, infections<br>• needs further evaluation |
| extreme fatigue | having more difficulty with the activity than others | Severe AMS<br>HAPE<br>HACE | • check breathing and if rapid at rest, treat for HAPE<br>• check tandem walking and if poor, treat for HACE<br>• do not raise sleeping altitude |
| ataxia | lack of coordination; determine by the tandem walking test | Severe AMS<br>HACE | • descend<br>• oxygen<br>• hyperbaric bag<br>• dexamethasone |
| altered mental status | an alteration in intellectual functioning, with emotional, attitudinal, psychologic and personality aspects | Severe AMS<br>HACE | • descend<br>• oxygen<br>• hyperbaric bag<br>• dexamethasone |
| diarrhea | | travelers' diarrhea | • hydrate<br>• antibiotic<br>• consider rest day |
| lack of appetite | | AMS, HAPE, HACE, other | • look for symptoms of other illnesses |
| feeling faint | a very difficult complaint to analyze since people can mean almost anything by it | almost any condition | • check ability to concentrate and do simple math.<br>• check tandem walking<br>• give fluids if light-headed<br>• consider a rest day |

**Table 2 Altitude Illness**

| Altitude Illnesses | How Common (approx. percentage) trekkers to Everest Base Camp | climbers on Mount Rainier | climbers on Mount McKinley | Common Altitude of Occurrence (feet/meters) | Common Symptoms | Treatment | Other Treatment | Mortality Rate |
|---|---|---|---|---|---|---|---|---|
| **Acute Mountain Sickness (AMS)** | | | | | | | | |
| Mild | 50 | 70 | 65 | 10,000/3,050 | like a hangover | don't raise sleeping altitude | simple pain medicines, acetazolamide | 0 |
| Severe | 2 | 0 | 2 to 4 | 15,000/4,575 | difficulty coordinating | descend immediately | hyperbaric bag, oxygen, acetazolamide dexamethasone | low if treated |
| **High Altitude Pulmonary Edema (HAPE)** | 1 to 2 | 0 | 3 | 14,000/4,270 | extreme shortness of breath | descend immediately | hyperbaric bag, nifedipine oxygen | low if treated quickly |
| **High Altitude Cerebral Edema (HACE)** | 0.05 | 0 | 0.5 | 15,000/4,575 | poor coordination progresses to extreme lethargy and coma | give dexamethasone, descend immediately | hyperbaric bag oxygen | higher than for HAPE |

## Table 3 High Altitude Drugs

| Name | Use | Form | Dose | How Often | Common Side Effects | Notes |
|------|-----|------|------|-----------|---------------------|-------|
| oxygen | treatment of all forms of altitude illness | cylinders by mask, or nasal prongs | 1 to 12 liters a minute; begin with 6 liters in serious problems | continuously | none in the mountain setting except possibly dry mucous membranes | delivery units with tight-fitting masks and a reservoir bag |
| acetazolamide | prevention of AMS | 250 mg tablet | 1/2 tablet | twice a day or at bedtime | increased urine output tingling of lips and extremities | do not give if allergic to sulfa drugs |
| | treatment of AMS | | 1 tablet | twice at day for treatment | | |
| nifedipine | treatment of HAPE | 10 mg capsule (pricked many times with a pin) | 1 capsule chewed and then swallowed | repeat in 15 minutes | lowering of blood pressure | see text for protocol details; follow with prevention dose |
| | prevention and treatment of HAPE | 20 mg slow-release capsule (Adalat®) | 1 capsule swallowed | every 6 hours | lowering of blood pressure | see text for protocol details |
| | | 30 mg extended release tablet (Procardia XL®) | 1 or 2 tablets | daily | ankle swelling is commonly seen in lowlanders | |
| dexamethasone | treatment of Severe AMS and HACE | 4 mg tablets | 1 tablet | every 6 hours | emotional problems especially after stopping the drug; depression and euphoria reported while taking it | stop after problem has resolved |
| furosemide (frusemide) | treatment of peripheral edema | 40 mg tablets | 1/2 to 1 tablet | once a day | can cause fainting if taken while dehydrated | stop after edema has resolved; eat potassium (bananas, pigmented fruits); drink plenty of liquids |

# Bibliography

Asterisks (*) mark items recommended for non-medical readers.

Bezruchka, S. (1992). "High altitude medicine." Med Clin North Am 76(6): 1481-97.

*Bezruchka, S. (1999). *The Pocket Doctor: Your Ticket to Good Health While Traveling.* Seattle, The Mountaineers.

*Grissom, C. K. (1993). "Medical Therapy of High Altitude Illness." American Alpine Journal 35(67): 118-123.

Grissom, C. K., R. C. Roach, et al. (1992). "Acetazolamide in the treatment of acute mountain sickness: clinical efficacy and effect on gas exchange." Ann Intern Med 116(6): 461-5.

*Hackett, P. H. (1980). *Mountain Sickness: Prevention, Recognition and Treatment.* New York, American Alpine Club.

Hackett, P. H., R. C. Roach, et al. (1992). "The effect of vasodilators on pulmonary hemodynamics in high altitude pulmonary edema: a comparison." Int J Sports Med 13 (Supp 1): S68-S71.

*Houston, C. (1998). *Going Higher: Oxygen, Man, and Mountains.* Seattle: The Mountaineers.

Hultgren, Herbert. *High Altitude Medicine.* Stanford: Hultgren Publications, 1997. Order from (650) 857-9574, Fax (650) 493-4225, hultgren@highaltitudemedicine.com.

Kayser, B. (1991). "Acute mountain sickness in western tourists around the Thorong pass (5400 m) in Nepal." Jr Wild Med 2: 110-117.

Levine, B. D., J. Stray-Gundersen (1995). "Exercise at high altitudes." in *Current Therapy in Sports Medicine,* J.S. Torg and R.J. Shephard, St. Louis, Mosby.

Oelz, O., M. Maggiorini, et al. (1992). "Prevention and treatment of high altitude pulmonary edema by a calcium channel blocker." Int J Sports Med 13 (Supp 1): S65-S68.

Pollard, A.J., D.R. Murdoch. *The High Altitude Medicine Handbook.* Oxford: Radcliffe Medical Press, 1997.

Shlim, D. R. and J. Gallie (1992). "The causes of death among trekkers in Nepal." Int J Sports Med 13 (Supp 1): S74-S76.

# Index

# Notes

# Notes

# About the Author

Stephen Bezruchka has lived at altitude and ascended to extreme altitudes. He has climbed in Canada, the United States, China, Pakistan, and Nepal. Educated at Harvard, Stanford, and Johns Hopkins universities and at the University of Toronto, he is a board-certified emergency medicine specialist and teaches in the School of Public Health and Community Medicine of the University of Washington. He tries to disseminate information on the relationship between income distribution and the health of populations. He has provided health care in a remote region of Nepal, has collaborated with that government to turn a rural district hospital into a teaching hospital for Nepali doctors, and now works to improve surgical services in remote district hospitals there. He is the author of *The Pocket Doctor, Trekking in Nepal: A Traveler's Guide*, and *Nepali for Trekkers*. He is a member of the American Alpine Club, the Alpine Club of Canada, the UIAA (Union International des Associations d'Alpinism) Medical Commission, and the Wilderness Medical Society. He qualified to join the Supine Alpine Club, whose bylaws require members to have suffered from AML (Acute Mountain Lassitude), TT (Terminal Torpor), and HAFE.